Complexity in Health Care

Steven A. Frankel · Steven D. Thurber
James A. Bourgeois

Complexity in Health Care

A Paradigm Shift for Clinical Practice

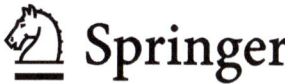 Springer

Steven A. Frankel, M.D.
Department of Psychiatry
and Behavioral Sciences
University of Minnesota School
of Medicine
Minneapolis, MN, USA

Steven D. Thurber, Ph.D.
Department of Psychiatry
and Behavioral Sciences
University of Minnesota School
of Medicine
Minneapolis, MN, USA

James A. Bourgeois, O.D., M.D.
Department of Psychiatry
and Behavioral Sciences
UC Davis Medical Center
University of California, Davis
Sacramento, CA, USA

ISBN 978-3-031-14948-1   ISBN 978-3-031-14949-8   (eBook)
https://doi.org/10.1007/978-3-031-14949-8

This Springer imprint is published by the registered company Springer Nature Switzerland AG
The registered company address is: Gewerbestrasse 11, 6330 Cham, Switzerland

This book is dedicated to Philip Erdberg, Ph.D., who was a dear friend and a towering presence in the mental health field. Phil died on April 23, 2023. Phil worked closely with Steve Frankel for more than 40 years. Phil authored three notable books and multiple professional papers. He was a pioneer in the development of the Rorschach Psychological Assessment, bringing it to its contemporary form as the R-PAS Psychological Assessment. It would be hard to overstate the power of Phil's thinking. His intellectual prowess and versatility were perhaps best illustrated when Phil, who grew up in Oklahoma, delivered at least one of his international lectures entirely in Spanish. Phil's brilliance was paralleled by his integrity. Along with George Washington of cherry tree fame, it is easy to imagine Phil saying,
"I have never told a lie."

Phil was a visionary in the area of clinical complexity. The R-PAS represents a consolidation of myriad psychological dimensions, with meticulous attention to how each contributes to the overall psychological status of a patient. It is easy to see how his subject squares with our focus on clinical complexity. There are few people who we believe have appreciated the multifaceted nature of each clinical situation as well as Phil did.

Personal Dedications:

Steven A. Frankel: *is grateful for the presence of his wife. Diane Engelman and the support of his remarkable adult children Peter and Cara as well as their children Nathan and Ayla.*

Steven D. Thurber: *to my adult children, David, Janean, and Eric, for being a source of pride and inspiration.*

James A. Bourgeois *thanks his family for their unwavering support. His wife, Kathleen M. Ayers, Psy.D., specializes in the psychotherapy of patients with chronic systemic illness. His son, Emile W. Ayers Bourgeois, M.B.A., is a mechanical engineer for Siemens. His daughter, Germaine A. Ayers Bourgeois, suffers from the NBIA Disorder MPAN. She previously worked at a remarkable facility for special needs adults, Brookwood in Georgetown (brookwoodingeorgetown.org) near our previous home in Georgetown Texas (suburban Austin).*

We are of course grateful to the staff at the New York office of Springer Publishing and to Eugenia Judson our talented developmental editor at the Springer office in

Chennai India for their support and guidance. Melanie Zerah, our managing editor, has been outstanding in her availability and her openness to our ideas. She has indeed been a continual inspiration as we have created this book. Special thanks go to our computer guru, Karl Krause. He is not only a brilliant technician, but his tireless guidance remained ever present throughout the rigors of creating and refining this book. Karl is the kind of friend that we could only have hoped for. Steady, smart, generous, and thoroughly genuine.

Foreword

Reading *Complexity in Health Care: A Paradigm Shift for Clinical Practice,* I frequently thought back to a patient I saw as a young psychiatrist. The resident in the emergency department (ED) called me to see a "psychotic patient" whom the family brought in. The resident admitted that he hardly saw the need to involve me in "a straightforward psychosis." Having completed the exam and routine labs, all of which were normal, he planned to transfer the patient to the local psychiatric hospital. However, hospital policy required a psychiatrist to sign off on the transfer, hence the call. Being a busy day, I did not put this high on my priority list and arrived at the ED a considerable time later to sign off on this reportedly simple patient.

I'm guessing you can see what I did not suspect then—what I found was anything but simple. For starters, the patient could not speak English, only Vietnamese, as did most of her family. All communication had been through a daughter, who did not live with the patient. Furthermore, the patient was not cooperative with any exam—she was constantly getting up and walking around the room while rapidly talking to staff, seemingly unaware that no one but her family could understand her.

I first insisted that we call for a professional interpreter, which irritated the hurried resident as this meant we had to call one in, thus delaying the transfer. While waiting, I talked with the daughter. She maintained that her 45-year-old mother had never experienced anything like this, nor had her family. Her mother had emigrated from Vietnam two years earlier to join her children in the USA. She suspected that her mother was a victim of past abuse, both physically and sexually. However, the family never discussed this. The daughter visited daily and, on this day, found her mother on the floor of her room. Oddly, her father had not thought this unusual, but she convinced him to help her bring the mother to the ED.

When I interviewed the patient, it was challenging to make sense of the interpretation, particularly after I asked the newly arrived interpreter to stop paraphrasing and tell me verbatim what the patient said. What I found curious was that the patient was complaining of terrible headaches and vague references to being assaulted, possibly by her husband.

Ultimately, I told the ED resident we needed more information, starting with brain imaging. The resident was exasperated, saying that the neurological examination was normal and there was no indication for such a test. I avoided wondering out loud how one could do a complete neuro exam on a constantly moving patient. The ED resident argued with me, saying the psychiatric hospital had already accepted the patient for admission, all they needed was my signature, and any further workup could happen there. Behind this was the understandable fear that if we delayed too long, we would lose the bed, and the patient could remain in the ED for days.

I was getting nowhere with the resident, but fortunately, the Chief of Emergency Medicine walked by. He knew me and seemed to like me, and after the resident related my "unreasonable demand," he shrugged and said if I thought it necessary, they should do it. He suggested a Computerized Tomography (CT) scan to rule out anything acute, as it seemed unlikely the patient would remain cooperative with an MRI, which was the wisest step.

Knowing this would take time, I went off to take care of the rest of my long to-do list. Several hours passed, and I was confused that I had not heard back from the ED. Had they just bypassed me and transferred the patient? I went back to the ED, and when I asked the chief whether I should start the transfer, he smiled wryly and said no; the patient had been quickly whisked off to neurosurgery for an emergency craniotomy after the CT revealed an acute bleed in her brain. He patted my shoulder, saying that was a pretty good pickup up, "especially for a shrink."

My first reaction was a feeling of triumph. I had stood my ground—indeed, this seemed a moment for quiet celebration. Nevertheless, my subsequent reaction was intense anxiety. There were plenty of patients deemed routine whom I had quickly sent to the psychiatric hospital. So how did I know, this time, to take a pause? Sure there was a communication barrier, but in the multicultural environment I worked, that was not unusual. Why did I push?

There were clues in the history, headaches, and observable behaviors, but all were nonspecific and otherwise explainable. Ultimately I did not know. It was just a "gut feeling" that something was not right. I ran it by peers who would shrug and say, "clinical wisdom."

All this is a long way to say that I wish I had this book back then.

I mainly have known Drs. Frankel and Thurber from their written works and reputation. Dr. Frankel has written several previous works on treating complex patients and the psychotherapeutic process. Years ago, I even reviewed his excellent book *Comprehensive Care for Complex Patients: The Medical-Psychiatric Coordinating Physician Model*, coauthored by Dr. Bourgeois and Philip Erdberg. I found it to be an excellent meditation on the body-mind interface and the role of doctors in modern medicine. Dr. Thurber, I mainly know through his publications on delirium—I was particularly intrigued by a 2008 study he participated in showing that many general hospital consultations to the psychiatry service are unrecognized delirium—a particular pet peeve of mine. Finally, I know Dr. Bourgeois the best, as he is a leading figure in the field of Consultation-Liaison Psychiatry. I have had the great pleasure of hearing him speak, serving on committees with him, reading his many scientific papers, and, most recently, briefly collaborating with him during his tenure as Chair of Psychiatry at the neighboring

Baylor Scott & White Health and Texas A&M University before his move to the west coast. I must admit, though, that despite admiring him for years, it was only recently, while reviewing his biography, that I discovered he was an optometrist as well as a psychiatrist!

Given my respect for this team, I was thrilled to be asked to write this preface, if only because that meant I would get an advanced copy of the book. So when you read this, you will find what I did—a tour de force examination of the clinical encounter and what the doctor-patient relationship actually means.

The early chapters may confuse one a bit. They are sometimes somewhat abstract summaries of various aspects of the scientific method as it applies to medicine. Although I found this part fascinating, as it was an articulate summary of the science behind the clinical studies we read, I began to wonder where this was all going. Indeed, I have heard presentations about the nature of complexity in medicine that has been entirely incomprehensible, at least to the practical-minded such as myself, and I started to worry. However, I need not have. The method behind their madness becomes apparent as they use this section as a foundation and apply the principles to patient care.

An example is their brilliant work organizing the many variables we encounter, grouping them into the easily measurable and the more elusive, all critical to understanding the patient. In this sense, the authors become master organizers, able to take all the things experienced clinicians intuitively understand and put them into a framework that is accessible and practical. Why is this important? Much like my anxiety about my "good pickup" with the patient, we cannot simply trust our guts all the time. Likewise, we cannot depend on doing something as complex as treating patients consistently if we do not understand how we do what we do.

However, the heart of the book is the fascinating case studies. Following in the tradition of the great clinicians: Freud, Charcot, Kraepelin, and more contemporaneously, Oliver Sacks and Glen Gabbard, these are not the bloodless cases we see in journals but artfully drawn verbal illustrations that not only acknowledge but revel in the many nooks and crannies we find when we come to know a patient deeply. They then use the clever technique of not only discussing the relevance of the case initially but repeatedly coming back to the case, adding details, and broadening their discussion of what this tells us about treating complex cases.

As Winston Churchill said, "*Out of intense complexities, intense simplicities emerge.*" We may not finish the book thinking that treating patients is exactly simple, but at least we will likely find comfort in their approach and begin to find complex patients more comprehensible. There are many lessons to take away from this book, more than I can or should mention here—to understand the book, you have to read it, preferably in the order it is written. Some takeaways for me include a broadening of the idea of what is a complex patient. Reflecting on my years as a geriatric and consultation-liaison psychiatrist and now in a leadership role at the Menninger Clinic, a hospital specializing in intense treatment, I cannot help but read this book and think that all patients are complex. The ones that are not are simply people we have not gotten to know very well. This fact is another important lesson: to treat patients, we must know them well. No matter how much we prefer to put patients into manageable categories and apply simple algorithms to treat them, genuine treatment comes when we join the patient in a relationship, tolerate our shortcomings, expend the time and energy to know the patient as best as we can, and join together toward a common goal. This is the lesson I have learned from my best mentors and teachers. Is this hard work? Of course, but there is no substitute for it. The payoff, of course, is that this hard work gives our work and our lives meaning. Rather than "burnout" (now becoming a cliché among medical doctors), we find joy in what we do. After reading this book, I now better understand why.

Senior Vice President & Chief of Staff,   Robert J. Boland, M.D.
The Menninger Clinic
Professor and Vice Chair,
Menninger Department of Psychiatry
and Behavioral Sciences
The Brown Foundation Endowed Chair in Psychiatry
Baylor College of Medicine
Houston, TX, USA

Preface

Premise of This Book

Patients individually comprise systems that are remarkably complicated, both structurally and functionally. Myriad components (variables) interact, continually reshaping each subsystem. Attempting to simplify a clinical situation through diagnoses and algorithms is attractive and necessary, but invariably leaves out details that matter for accurately understanding a patient. Additional variables may include demographics, medical information, social and cultural considerations, and individual patient traits such as resilience.

The patient system is not static. While usually moved by treatment in the direction of healing (health), all parts interact and remain influential. This fluidity helps to explain why it is so difficult to predict treatment outcomes. The treatment paradigm we advocate is based on this inherent complexity and dynamism. The building blocks of that model are variables that may include concrete factors such as symptoms and medications, subjective components such as attitudes that influence clinical activity, social factors, and nonhuman contributions such as mathematical and statistical assumptions.

It is tempting to seek a strictly mathematical, i.e., quantitative, method for organizing all these components and calculating the product of their interaction. Such methods might include multivariate statistics, factor analysis, or algorithms involved in machine learning and artificial intelligence as applied to clinical data. In our opinion these synthetic attempts, though laudable for what they can produce in clinical decisional support, will inevitably prove inadequate by themselves when applied to the human system. Humans are constantly in flux. Contributing factors may come into play rapidly and randomly, thereby keeping the system unstable.

Remaining is the human contribution to clinical work, broadly understood as clinical judgment. Perhaps surprisingly, clinical judgment has an excellent track record for guiding clinical work. However, relying on clinical judgment requires understanding its limits and maintaining the uncertainty required for trusting a subjective process. In addition, the more educated, informed, and "current" the clinician is, the better his or her judgment is likely to be.

Corte Madera, CA, USA   Steven A. Frankel, M.D.
Minneapolis, MN, USA   Steven D. Thurber, Ph.D.
Sacramento, CA, USA   James A. Bourgeois, O.D., M.D.

Contents

Part XVII   Conclusion, Clinching the Paradigm Shift

Part I

Guiding Principles

1

Introduction

In this book, we propose a paradigm shift for clinical practice. This model underscores the vast numbers of variables that are influential in clinical work. Included are those that tend to be undervalued or unappreciated. We also bring to light the full complexity of the clinical field consisting not just of an array of variables but their interactions as well.

New thinking in science tends to emerge the "hard way." Adherents to accepted viewpoints may tenaciously resist new ways of understanding and working. Disagreements over new ideas may become heated, even violent. Indeed, a scientist who opposes a prevailing theory or procedure needs to be careful to avoid being dismissed or ostracized. Thomas Kuhn eloquently described this stifling atmosphere, citing resistance originally encountered to Newtonian physics and quantum theory [1]. Richard Feynman, twentieth-century physicist, created groundbreaking work which was originally ridiculed for its alleged excessive "simplicity" [2]. It was similar for Albert Einstein whose special theory of relativity was originally dismissed as likely incorrect and nonetheless irrelevant [3].

This propensity to react against or reject what is new but inconsistent with established ideas has a long history in medicine and science. The intensity with which new ideas may be resisted is exemplified by the experience of the Hungarian physician, Ignaz Semmelweis [4]. In the mid-nineteenth century, prior to Louis Pasteur's contributions on the germ theory [5], Semmelweis worked in an obstetrical clinic in which physicians who delivered babies also performed autopsies. Semmelweis found that high rates of "childhood fever" could be reduced significantly if physicians removed "cadaverous particles" by washing their hands with a chlorinated lime solution before extending services to pregnant women. The simple handwashing recommendation, based on solid but *new* evidence, was soundly rejected by physicians for reasons related to disruption of the status quo.

© The Author(s), under exclusive license to Springer Nature Switzerland AG 2023
S. A. Frankel et al., *Complexity in Health Care*,
https://doi.org/10.1007/978-3-031-14949-8_1

The Origin of New Ideas in Clinical Practice

Where do new ideas come from? How often do they occur? Did you notice that the woman who checks your bag at the grocery store recalled your name after 5 years, when you only shopped at the store twice earlier? Perhaps she recalled your smile, or maybe it was something about the question you asked about her labored gait. How about Charles, my (SAF)[1] Down syndrome patient, who remembered our raucous teasing of each other who remembered our raucous teasing of each other a year previously and who skillfully taught me how to communicate with him. Charles had only limited use of language but was able to guide us. The point is that new, creative ideas may arise seemingly from nowhere. They percolate in the mind of the subject and may consolidate into new, even remarkable configurations, each with its own kernel of brilliance.

Inspiration for This Book

Surprising, in effect often remarkable, events like these were the inspiration for this book. We bring our experience, SAF's (Steven A. Frankel) in clinical work as a child-adolescent and general psychiatrist, ST's (Steven D. Thurber) in biostatistics and clinical psychology, and JAB's (James A. Bourgeois) in hospital-based academic consultation-liaison psychiatry, as formal background for the ideas we present. But we also bring our passion for new ideas and ultimately for shifting to new perspectives that may improve our clinical work. Standard clinical methods generally use algorithms as heuristics. Our goal is to improve clinical work without "losing" the patient through this summarizing of his or her medical-psychological-social history and simplifications of the clinical findings.

Clinical Complexity

Clinical situations are complex with contributions from (a) commonly understood, as well as (b) more obscure personal, social, and cultural sources. Clinical situations should be valued according to their contribution to outcome (healing, cure). Clinical judgments and actions, while they may be evidence-based, are often impressionistic. Some determinants will be partially included and emphasized as well as deemphasized or excluded by practitioners based on their opinions and experience. We assume that the clinical factors most likely to be bypassed or minimized by practitioners are those that are subjective in nature (e.g., personal, emotional), at least partially arising in the minds of the patient and clinician. For this book, our data will consist of (1) recorded clinical experience, (2) literature on the clinical process and its structure and complexity, and (3) research we have reviewed and conducted on diagnosis and treatment of challenging patients.

---

[1] The abbreviation "SAF" from this point will refer to co-author Steven A. Frankel.

References

1. Kuhn TS. The structure of scientific revolutions. In: The structure of scientific revolutions. 4th ed. Chicago: Chicago University Press; 2012.
2. Feynman RP. In: Feynman M, editor. The quotable Feynman: Princeton University press [internet]. Princeton, NJ: Princeton University Press; 2016. Available from:. https://doi.org/10.1515/9781400874231.
3. Albert Einstein's special theory of relativity: emergence (1905 and early interpretation) by Arthur I. Miller.
4. Semmelweis I. Aetiology, concept and prophylaxis of childbed fever. Madison, WI: University of Wisconsin Press; 1983.
5. Armentrout D, Armentrout P. Pasteur's contributions on the germ theory. Rourke Publishing; 2002.

Part II

The Clinical Situation

[Part Introduction: In this part of the book, we list the elements of the clinical situation. Our plan is to deconstruct its complexity prior to describing how its pieces work together. Virtually all clinical situations are complicated, albeit to varying degrees. They consist of numbers of variables contributed by the patient(s) and clinicians, and myriad technical features each of which is a clinical variable. These variables taken together constitute the "structure" of the case. But importantly that "structure" is dynamic, changing over time. We classify variables as "clinical" as they are brought into play for the purpose of treatment, i.e., the goal of healing.

The clinician is not just challenged to unravel this complicated situation but also to represent the patient accurately, including his or her "human" elements as represented by temperament and personal attitudes. What are the patient's essential needs, tolerances, preferences? Yet, there is even more to know about each patient. Does she have children? What is her financial status, her ethnicity? What are her attitudes about medical professionals. Does she believe in medicine, or even in science?

Beware! None of these factors are dispensable when trying to understand a patient. Just try to leave out a few and you are left with a gutted rendering of that person, not a living human being.

Traditionally a medical patient is subjected to an extensive workup that includes a mental status examination, in addition to a detailed past and present history, and an extensive "review of (organ) systems." The result even when this level of detail is available may still be an anemic version of the patient. Now add the multiplicity of problems, psychiatric and systemic medical, from which the patient suffers. Multiplicity may include systemic medical, psychiatric, social, financial, and lack of access to health providers.

From this description it seems logical that complex patients presenting with mixed medical-psychiatric disorders be managed with an ongoing collaborative approach delivered by a multispecialty team. Included may be a primary care physician, psychiatrist, and/or psychotherapists. One or more of the collaborating professionals may be a nurse practitioner and/or a physician's assistant.

Clearly, the clinical requirements for treating complex patients often exceed boundaries usually associated with care of a "systemic illness" and/or a "psychiatric disorder." For these patients an actively engaged case manager is likely to be an essential addition to the treatment team. The assistance provided by these practitioners include logistical help to the primary clinician(s). This function is invaluable for navigating a cumbersome health-care delivery system that is not designed to access and monitor customized multispecialty care.]

The "Clinical Situation": An Introduction to Its Structure and Complexity

2

Introduction

This chapter identifies the range of variables that comprise a clinical situation. These variables can reconfigure and interact. Each new configuration is a separate entity. These variables may be conveniently collected under a label such as "biopsychosocial." However, designations such as "biopsychosocial" are often not adequate for conveying the full (detailed) nature of a clinical situation. This chapter begins to elaborate the array of variables and their manifestations that clinicians may encounter when working with patients, especially complex patients.

Most clinical situations "up close" are quite complicated. Parts contribute and interrelate, comprising a "complex clinical field." In this book, we are interested in recognizing and working with the broad range of case-related variables that make up a clinical situation. Included are systemic medical, psychiatric, psychological, and cultural contributions and ways these interact and influence each other. Specifically emphasized are clinical variables that are hard to define and are at least partially subjective.

To date, we have written about work with complex patients and cases. In this volume, we embrace the broad clinical field, often focusing on clinical factors that are considered marginal in clinical work. Relevant also is the treater's and patient's personal influence on clinical work. We hold that without the full recognition of these often less acknowledged contributions, clinical work cannot be adequately understood. We will ultimately present a model (paradigm) for understanding and working with complex patients and cases.

In addition to drawing from the medical literature, this book also acknowledges contributions from the social sciences, including psychology, social work, and sociology. These contributions are manifold and for those who work with these patients incorporates a broad range of clinical situations. Adding substance to our work is research we have done or plan to undertake to identify factors associated with treatment of complex clinical situations and the associated complex patients.

© The Author(s), under exclusive license to Springer Nature Switzerland AG 2023
S. A. Frankel et al., *Complexity in Health Care*,
https://doi.org/10.1007/978-3-031-14949-8_2

Clinical Situations "Up Close"

There are few clinical situations that are not inherently complicated when looked at closely. Structurally, these situations may be quite different one from another. Some involve the treatment of complicated, "hard-to-treat" diseases. Other situations may be difficult to work with primarily because of personal and social challenges. In this book, we refer to the aggregate of these clinical situations as "clinically complex." Typically, medical patients labeled as "complex" have multiple acute and chronic diseases, comorbid psychiatric illness, *and* social problems.

These patients may, and usually do, require excess resources to treat. For their psychiatric comorbid illnesses, they may need psychiatric or other mental health treatment. For their social problems, they may require social work and/or other case management services. In this book, an expanded range of clinically relevant influences (clinical variables), including those that elude objectification, are considered. Informing our portrayal is the frequent experience of the clinician who becomes aware of the insufficiencies of his or her treatment model recognizing that unaccounted for factors are at work.

Roger Kathol has eloquently defined "health complexity" as "the interference with the achievement of expected or desired health and cost outcomes, due to the interaction of biological, psychological, social and health systems factors when patients are exposed to standard care delivered by their doctors" [1]. This definition is structurally and operationally different from our own definition of health complexity. Nonetheless, it underscores the disparate nature of complex health situations, their character defined according to a diverse set of criteria: personal, cultural, and institutional. Added is the fact that the general medical and behavioral health-care delivery systems are for the most part separated administratively, increasing the challenges in delivering integrated care to these complex patients.

Because of the multiplicity and chronicity of their illnesses, complex patients usually require excess resources beyond "usual care." For their psychiatric comorbid illnesses, they need psychiatric or other mental health treatment, and for their social problems require social work and/or other case management services. In this book, an expansive range of clinically relevant influences (clinical variables), including those that elude simple objectification, are considered. Informing our portrayal is the frequent experience of the clinician who becomes aware of the insufficiencies of his or her treatment model recognizing that unaccounted for factors are at work.

Most primary and specialty general medical care, and psychiatric and other behavioral health-care models are disconnected fiscally. Compensation for psychiatric and behavioral health care is frequently subject to different standards and regulations than those for general medical care. Inter-professional communication between general medicine and psychiatry is often poor due to privacy concerns. As an example, sharing of psychotherapy and substance abuse treatment notes and data is subject to specific and often severe restrictions.

Case Managers

Management of a complex clinical case is difficult enough. Here we add the central position that case managers have in this process. Case managers can be essential for care planning and execution. A case manager follows a patient closely, communicates with family, and assesses progress using qualitative and quantitative measures. Case managers may initially be certified in nursing, social work, or have a bachelor's degree in psychology. Added is specialized training and certification through their own professional organization, e.g., Case Management Society of America. They are also required to have a set number of years of work experience. Case managers provide logistical and supportive assistance to patients for coordinating clinical care and navigating an often cumbersome health-care system. This function includes providing facilitated access to specialty physicians and encouragement of communication among treating and consulting physicians. Similarly, physician assistants and nurse practitioners (who also may share the function of case managers) may be responsible for elements of primary care management and overall care coordination of these patients. Because of the complexity of the clinical situations to which we refer, and the scarcity and expense of physician's time, these allied health-care personnel are essential for supporting and enhancing the medical care of complex patients.

Note that case managers do not replace physicians. They do not write medical orders. Instead, they carry out the following responsibilities:

- Screening to see if case management services are needed
- Assessing
- Risk evaluation
- Planning
- Implementing
- Outcome evaluation

In summary, case management is a collaborative process of assessment, planning, facilitation, care coordination, evaluation, and advocacy for the comprehensive health needs of patients and families. Case managers help to identify appropriate providers and facilities throughout a continuum of medically related services.

Our Publications and Research on Clinical Complexity

Clinical complexity is an area that has generated much contemporary interest. "Comprehensive," "collaborative," and "integrated" care have become popular topics in the medical literature and refer to simultaneous presence of multiple clinical variables. Many of these models provide structures for the delivery of psychiatric and other mental health services in the general medical setting, with regular reciprocal communication between medical and behavioral health clinicians included. When needed, case management services can and often should be added to this range of clinical interventions.

"Interpersonal" and "intersubjective" treatment models have been frequent topics in the clinical literature. They generally refer to the interplay of personal variables encountered in treatment. Our goal in this book is to bring this full range of complexity to the attention of clinicians of various clinical disciplines and "unpack" ways of managing it. We know of no other volume dedicated to elucidating the full range of contributing clinical variables. Included are those variables that while not typically credited as making important contributions to clinical outcome actually do.

Regarding our research in the area of clinical complexity, we are completing a research project to validate the "Intermed Self-Assessment" evaluation (IMSA) using data from a socioeconomically burdened population of HIV-positive patients and have embarked on a project to create a screening tool for the identification of at-risk complex patients who require a full clinical assessment of their needs using the extensive observer rated VB ICM-CAG (Value-Based Integrated Case Management-Complexity Assessment Grid).

This book includes and goes beyond the following topics:

- The structure and nature of the clinical field, its components, and how these evolve over time
- The definition and management of clinical complexity, including organizing and working with complex clinical presentations
- Detailed examples of complex cases
- Our research on understanding and managing complex clinical situations
- It touches on advanced means for working with clinically complex situations involving "big data," machine learning, and/or artificial intelligence
- Within the category of elusive variables, we explore societal issues including cultural influences
- The culture of medicine and its preference for heuristic approaches to clinical detail

This book provides a resource for unpacking (deconstructing) complex clinical situations to discover their nature and dynamics.

Our Definition of Clinical Complexity

We end this chapter with our own, admittedly broad, definition of clinical complexity. Complex clinical situations are simply those that are not fully understandable or treatable by established clinical means, whether medical, psychotherapeutic, pharmacological, environmental change, or a combination of these modalities. A convenient "marker" of a complex patient is excessive and often nonproductive utilization of clinical services beyond that required by a "typical" patient (or, if you will, a "routine" patient). The objective of the investigative approaches detailed in this book is to "unpack" such complex clinical situations so they can be understood and productively worked with clinically. The goal is to create a unified approach (new paradigm or paradigm shift) for working with these inherently irregular situations. The following references are intended to give the reader an introduction to the endless dimensions of clinical complexity.

This and the next chapter provide both static and dynamic pictures of how the clinical situation is structured and works.

Reference

1. Kathol RG, Andrew RL, Squire M, Dehnel PJ. The integrated case management manual: value-based assistance to complex medical and behavioral health patients. 2nd ed. Basel: Springer; 2018.

Further Reading:

Our Publications on Patient Complexity

Frankel S, Bourgeois J, Erdberg P. Comprehensive care for complex patients: the medical-psychiatric coordinating physician model. Cambridge University Press; 2013.

Frankel S, Bourgeois J, Ghidoni A, Piemonte C, Paderni S, Ferarri S. Progress with the INTERMED Self-Assessment (IMSA) Study: from European to international. J Psychosom Res. 2014;76:503.

Frankel S, Bourgeois J. The medical-psychiatric coordinating physician-led model: team-based treatment for complex patients. Psychosomatics. 2014;55(4):333–42.

Frankel S. Evidence from within: a paradigm for clinical practice. Rowman and Littlefield; 2008.

Frankel S. Hidden faults: resolving therapeutic disjunctions. New York: The Psychosocial Press; 2000.

Frankel S. Intricate engagements: the collaborative basis of therapeutic change. Jason Aronson Inc; 1995.

Frankel S. Making psychotherapy work, collaborating effectively with your patient. The Psychosocial Press; 2007.

Heiligenberg M, Frankel SA, Caarls PJ, Zepf R, Boenink AD, Latour CHM. The validity of the INTERMED self-assessment questionnaire in HIV-infected patients in the USA. In: Heiligenberg M, (submitted for publication).

Kishi Y, Hazama Y, Komagata Y, Ishizuka M, Karube M, Takahashi J, Thurber S. Validity of the INTERMED complexity instrument with older patients in a Japanese general hospital. Asian Acad Res J. 2016;3:224–34.

Kishi Y, Takumi I, Yamamoto H, Ishimaru T, Thurber S. Patient complexity, depression, and quality of life in patients with epilepsy at an epilepsy center in Japan. Epilepsia Open. 2022;7(3):414–21. https://doi.org/10.1002/epi4.12614.

Meller W, Specker S, Schultz P, Kishi Y, Thurber S, Kathol R. Using the INTERMED complexity instrument for a retrospective analysis of patients presenting with medical illness, substance use disorder, and other psychiatric illnesses. Ann Clin Psychiatry. 2015;27(1):38–43.

Thurber S, Wilson A, Realmuto G, Specker S. The relationship between the INTERMED patient complexity instrument and level of care utilization system (LOCUS). Int J Psychiatry Clin Pract. 2018;22:80–2.

Variables

3

Introduction

The variables that comprise the clinical situation are not static. They interact in complicated ways and change over time. Moreover, there are variables that may barely be considered relevant to a clinical situation and nonetheless are influential and affect clinical outcome [1]. In addition to recognizing the influence of these less acknowledged clinical variables, awareness of and preparation for variable change, emergence of new variables, and variable interactions all confront a clinician working with patient complexity. There are several categories of clinical variables. For example, "#1" (conventional) variables and "#2" (elusive, abstract) variables are defined by us in this chapter and elaborated throughout the book.

The clinical field has an array of components. Some are fixed and others change with shifts in the patient's clinical condition. Added are clinical and personal resources, the sufficiency and availability of which may vary during treatment. In this chapter, we separate conventional, clearly defined clinical variables (we call these "#1" variables) from those that are harder to pin down descriptively and operationally (designated by us as "#2" variables).

Variables Constituting the Clinical Field

This chapter provides both static and dynamic pictures of how the clinical situation is structured and works. What is meant by the "clinical field?" We are obviously talking about the context (time and place) in which clinical work takes place. OK, but how is one facet of the treatment conceptually separated from other parts that are occurring simultaneously? I intend to treat an infectious illness with an antibiotic, but what if the patient is *also* being treated for liver disease and/or a major depressive disorder?

Unless you clearly map out your clinical operation, you risk losing your way. As implied in the last chapter, complex clinical situations consist of many, often

© The Author(s), under exclusive license to Springer Nature Switzerland AG 2023
S. A. Frankel et al., *Complexity in Health Care*,
https://doi.org/10.1007/978-3-031-14949-8_3

disparate, variables (symptoms, illnesses, procedures), e.g., rheumatic heart disease and major depressive disorder, each with different treatment requirements and influences on outcome. A hypothetical composite clinical field could contain a set of autoimmune findings and a depressive disorder. That patient would need attention by a primary care physician *and* a psychiatrist.

The Clinical Field: Its Structure

The following list of clinical variables and their sources is representative. The point is that the clinical field is flooded with content (variables) that are both physical and exist in the mind of the patient and/or clinician and is plagued by change as treatment evolves.

- **Examples of sources of clinically relevant factors, any, or all of which can be included in a single clinical situation**:
  - Biology, e.g., genetics, biochemistry, physiology.
  - Human development, e.g., physiological, psychological
  - Psychology, e.g., cognitive capabilities, emotional development
  - Social development
  - Personal and social sources including family and community
- **Dynamic factors**, a separate perspective that focuses on shifts within the clinical operation rather than its structure (otherwise labeled "dynamic complexity"). The clinical situation continually changes:
  - In response to biological influences
  - In response to life changes
  - Through subjective shifts including changes in the patient and practitioner as well as the patient's physical (medical) conditions that affect his or her sense of well-being, e.g., medication side effects, effects of illness on mood
  - Through changes in the patient's environment, including changes in the patient's living conditions, changes in key participants in the patient's life, medical treatments, and changes in that person's financial situation
- **Variables representing contributions from practitioner(s)**
  - Included are clinician's capabilities (training, skills), formal objectives, theoretical orientation, and biases.

Types of Variables

Not all clinical variables are easy to define or measure. In this book, we refer to those that can be clearly defined with referents in the physical world as "#1" variables. In contrast, failure to include variables that are imprecise and subjective or have an emotional correlate in a clinical formulation (throughout the book, we call these "#2" variables) often deprives the clinical situation of its full breadth and meaning. Examples of such variables include motivation, determination, pleasure, and anxiety. This omission would be ironic since these variables are ubiquitous in clinical work and invariably contribute, often heavily, to the treatment situation.

A clinical model without "#2" variables included in proportion to their influence on clinical outcome is necessarily insufficient. In this book, we will endeavor to characterize "#2" variables and identify ways these affect clinical work and its outcome. This book uses clinical examples and available research (including our own) to discover which variables are at work in specific clinical situations and to ascertain the impact of each on outcome. We call our method for identifying these variables the "empirical-collaborative" method.

Patients described in this book (myriad case examples are presented throughout the book) were seen adjunctively for separate or combined cognitive behavioral/ interpersonal psychotherapy, generally for one or two 30–50 minute meetings per week. The frequency and length of these sessions varied in accordance with symptom severity and tenacity. These patients were each being managed for systemic medical illness, most often chronic, and/or psychiatric illness. Cognitive behavioral and interpersonal psychotherapy (often combined) have been shown to provide symptom relief, bolster coping skills, and contribute to meaningful character change [2].

Beyond the essential role of consultation to ascertain psychiatric comorbidity (often multi-morbidity) impacting systemic medical illness, psychotherapy can be an important aspect of ongoing clinical management of complex patients [3]. The role of psychotherapy in this context is synergistic with the essential place for somatic psychiatric interventions, e.g., psychotropic medications, or neuromodulation, in managing specific psychiatric syndromes.

Abstract Variables

As we incorporate "#2" variables into our thinking, it should be beneficial to further explore what we mean when we refer to a concept as "abstract," i.e., "#2" variables as *harder to grasp* than "#1" variables which have discrete referents in the physical world. Are concrete and abstract variables interchangeable? Is there a process for making abstract designations more concrete and understandable? To accomplish this goal, we will use the abstract concept "intelligence."

The Process of Moving from the Abstract to the Concrete

How can an abstract, e.g., "#2" concept (variable), be made concrete? As an example, we will endeavor to create a measurable definition for the abstract term "intelligence." Intelligence refers to the capacity to act purposely, think rationally, and deal effectively with the environment. This essential step in constructing a specific "#1" variable definition from one that is indefinite, i.e., "#2" is called "construct explication." To accomplish this task, we search for explicit reference points for the term intelligence, e.g., scores on validated intelligence tests. In conducting this effort, we are admonished to "act purposely," "think rationally," and "deal effectively with the environment." Traversing a maze from start to finish via a series of complicated pathways is another example of purposeful behavior.

Now, in a methodical way, we have taken the familiar word "intelligence" and provided specific referents, building toward a precise definition. We now have referents that can be specified to "concretize" our abstract term "intelligence." Of note, many clinical variables like intelligence are afflicted with some ambiguity. They cannot be fully pinned down as to their specific referents and the way they may connect with other variables involved in diagnosis and treatment. The process of developing reliable definitions for clinical phenomena is of particular interest to us for operationalizing our clinical work.

Summary

The "takeaway" at this point is that there is no such thing as true simplicity within the clinical field. Its content consists of an uncountable number of variables. The clinical field is in constant motion based on change created through treatment and from the patient's social situation and biology. Our goal in future chapters will be to find ways to unpack this complexity so it remains as true to life as possible, not just manageable conceptually.

References

1. Jennissen S, Huber J, Erenthal JC. Association between insight and outcome of psychotherapy: systematic review and meta-analysis. Am J Psychiatr. 2018;175:961–9.
2. Markowitz JC, Weissman MM. Interpersonal psychotherapy, principles and applications. World Psychiatry. 2004;3(3):136–9.
3. Thomason TC. The trend toward evidence-based practice and the future of psychotherapy. Am J Psychother. 2010;64(1):29–38.

Further Reading

The Complexity of Clinical Judgment

Bonachela JA. Natural complexity: a modeling handbook. Princeton, NJ: Princeton University Press; 2017.
Charbonneau P. Primers in complex systems. Princeton (New Jersey): Princeton University Press, 2017. Q Rev Biol [Internet]. 2019;94(3):289–90.
Fink W, Lipatov V, Konitzer M. Diagnoses by general practitioners: accuracy and reliability. Int J Forecast. 2009;25(4):784–93.
Green LA, Fryer GE Jr, Yawn BP, Lanier D, Dovey SM. The ecology of medical care revisited. N Engl J Med [Internet]. 2001;344(26):2021–5. https://doi.org/10.1056/NEJM200106283442611.
Greenberg WKW. The environmental science of medical care. N Engl J Med. 1961.

Kienle GS, Kiene H. Clinical judgement and the medical profession: clinical judgement and medical profession. J Eval Clin Pract [Internet]. 2011;17(4):621–7.

Rosenberg CE. The tyranny of diagnoses: specific entities and individual experience. Milbank Q. 2002;80(2):237–60.

Sturmberg JP, Martin CM. The dynamics of health care reform--learning from a complex adaptive systems theoretical perspective. Nonlinear Dynamics Psychol Life Sci. 2010;14(4):525–40.

White KL, Williams TF, Greenberg BG. The ecology of medical care. Engl J Med [Internet]. 1961;265(18):885–92. https://doi.org/10.1056/nejm196111022651805.

The Following Readings Illustrate the Variety of Uses of the Concept "Clinical Complexity"

Croicu C, Chwastiak L, Katon W. Approach to the patient with multiple somatic symptoms. Med Clin North Am [Internet]. 2014;98(5):1079–95. https://doi.org/10.1016/j.mcna.2014.06.007.

Kathol RG, Andrew RL, Squire M, Dehnel PJ. Care plan development, barrier reversal, patient-centered ICM performance, graduation, and outcome analysis. In: The integrated case management manual. Cham: Springer; 2018. p. 191–206.

Kathol RG, Kathol MH. The need for biomedically and contextually sound care plans in complex patients. Ann Intern Med [Internet]. 2010;153(9):619–20; author reply 620. https://doi.org/1 0.7326/0003-4819-153-9-201011020-00018.

McGregor M, Lin EHB, Katon WJ. TEAMcare: an integrated multicondition collaborative care program for chronic illnesses and depression. J Ambul Care Manage [Internet]. 2011;34(2):152–62. https://doi.org/10.1097/JAC.0b013e31820ef6a4.

Part III

Technical Considerations

The main author for this part is Steven D. Thurber, Ph.D.

[Part Introduction: In this extensive part of the book, we discuss the formal, mathematical and statistical principles, underlying the paradigm shift we have formulated.

The paradigm we arrive at in this volume represents a form of scientific "emergence." The term emergence refers to a "whole" that derives from the interaction of subcomponents. The whole that emerges is unlike any of the individual parts. As a simple example, when the chemical element "hydrogen" interacts with the element "oxygen," there can be an emergence of the compound "water."

The emergence of the paradigm we present was the result of the authors' integration of scientific knowledge and clinical experience. In particular, this clinical model was influenced by scientific epistemology, including measurement and advanced statistics, theoretical modeling, clinical decision-making, cognitive biases, the investigations of the "awe" phenomena, and recent data on patient complexity, including that associated with the epigenome.

These creative paradigmatic influences will be interwoven in chapters throughout the text. This section of the book, as a departure from the clinical illustrations that populate the rest of the book, presents the foundations of clinical research, the technical background for the clinical-scientific principles we evolve and describe. We summarize the major technical foundations of a paradigm shift that eventuates in what may be a new clinical paradigm, with references to supporting scientific literature.]

Technical Principles of the Paradigm Shift We Adopt

4

Introduction

In this chapter, we present a brief history of science, its philosophical underpinnings (epistemology), and the fundamental components of the scientific method. A prime mover of scientific progress is measurement. Once a phenomenon of interest has been quantified, the powerful tools of mathematics can be implemented via statistical procedures. Some important statistical techniques found in medical and behavioral (psychiatric) science studies are presented. The chapter ends with a discussion of procedures for organizing measured, reliable, and valid scientific data into a theoretical model to guide clinical understanding of patients with biopsychosocial complexities, the foundations of our paradigm shift.

The paradigm shift we arrive at in this volume represents a form of scientific "emergence." The term emergence refers to a "whole" that derives from the interaction of its subcomponents. The whole that emerges may be unlike any of its component parts. As a simple example, when the chemical element hydrogen interacts with a different chemical element, e.g. oxygen, the resulting "whole," the liquid, water, has characteristics different from either component element.

The emergence of the paradigm we present occurred for us as the result of the integration of scientific knowledge and clinical experience. In particular, the clinical model that resulted was influenced by scientific epistemology, including measurement and advanced statistics, theoretical modeling, clinical decision-making, cognitive biases, the investigations of the "awe" phenomena, and recent data on patient complexity including that associated with the epigenome.

These creative paradigmatic influences will be interwoven in chapters throughout the text. This chapter of the book, as a departure from the clinical illustrations that populate the rest of the book, presents the technical background for the clinical-scientific principles we evolve. We summarize the major technical foundations of this paradigm shift together with supporting references to the scientific literature.

S. A. Frankel et al., *Complexity in Health Care*,
https://doi.org/10.1007/978-3-031-14949-8_4

Science, Measurement, and Statistics

In varying degrees, clinicians have a supply of information and skills for therapeutic interactions with patients. These contributions are based on formal training as well as clinical experience. Typically, this education incorporates instruction in the scientific method and exposure to relevant research. This chapter will provide a review of foundational aspects of these methods and their use for identification of variables making up the clinical situation and their interactions.

Science

On November 28, 1660, "science" officially began with the establishment of the Royal Society of London. Some of the notable persons involved include famous names such as Wren, Newton, and Boyle. The Royal Society began as a kind of revolt against the existing and dominant notions regarding what constitutes "truth," with science sometimes termed "the revolutionary epistemology." In the seventeenth century, prior to the emergence of science, there were two methods for establishing "truth." In "pessimistic epistemology," truth was the province of persons with power and authority. Thus, in this context, truth was defined as the utterances of Charles II, the King of England, or the authoritative writings of ecclesiastical leaders of the Church of England. The motto of the Royal Society was the Latin phrase *Nullius in verba* meaning "take nobody's word for it, virtually a statement nullifying truth via the pessimistic epistemology criterion" [1].

A second approach, inconsistent with the scientific, was termed "the optimistic epistemology." It is optimistic in the sense that truth was available to all persons capable of intuition and feeling. The truth of a proposition is how one feels about it. If it feels good, it has truth value" [2, 3].

The revolt against "truth" via authority and truth obtained via feeling led quite logically to a "revolutionary epistemology" or the scientific method. The simplistic notions of relying on the truth value of what someone in authority claims or upon one's emotional reactions were replaced by processes that were much more rigorous and time-consuming, the so-called scientific method. Below are likely familiar terms that comprise the revolutionary epistemology. We will discuss each in turn [4, 5].

1. Empirical
2. Measurement
3. Control
4. Null hypothesis
5. Falsifiability
6. Replication

These basic principles of science guide scientific investigations in medicine and the behavioral sciences, be they "N of 1," the study of the individual (the idiographic approach), or studies involving several persons (the nomothetic approach). A major point to be made is that the essential element of these principles is that they are calculated to reduce or eliminate human bias inherent in the optimistic and pessimistic propositions for truth-finding. As such, the scientific method can provide guidance for the rational thinking and actions of the clinician that at times may be quite apart from actual published scientific research.

What follows are the fundamental tenets of science:

Empirical

The word "empirical" refers to that which is observable. Instead of emotional reasoning or an authoritarian edict, the search for a scientific truth begins with what can be seen by any individual with intact sensory capacities, regardless of social status. A scientist can make inferences beyond the observable. Indeed, this is the job of the scientist (or clinician). But, at its core, a science must have a foundation of empirical facts. Analogously, at the core of effective clinical interventions are direct observations.

Measurement

Just because observations have occurred does not make them, *ad hoc,* "facts," What has been observed could be an illusion or some other type of faulty perception. If something exists, it can be quantified beyond zero. If it cannot be quantified in current time or potentially measured, it can be assumed that the phenomenon or variable of interest does not objectively exist.

Measurement has been the key to scientific advancements since the advent of the Royal Society. Examples include the measurement of the atom, the distance from earth to a celestial body, and a number representing one's general intelligence. Measurement refers to rules for the assignment of numbers to represent quantities. The rule for a multiple-choice achievement test, for instance, is typically one point (a number) for each correct alternative selection. As an example, for the previously discussed Value-Based Integrated Case Management (VB ICM-CAG) assessment instrument, trained raters are asked to respond to test items related to the chronicity of a physical symptom or presence of a plurality of symptoms according to the following rule:

0 = less than 3 months of duration
1 = more than 3 months
2 = a chronic condition
3 = several chronic conditions.

Measurement and Operational Definitions

One major goal in the behavioral sciences is to elucidate the nature of variables so they can be communicated in words and phrases. There are two fundamental definitional categories for indicating the group in which a word belongs (symbolizes), concrete or abstract. The former is "denotatively exact." These are words that specify some object in the environment that is tangible. You can literally point to or even touch the material thing, e.g., table, rug, car, cell phone, and telephone pole. These are "concrete" words.

In contrast, there are words in our language that are denotatively inexplicit or abstract. In this case, the exact nature of what is being denoted is at best imprecise or polysemous (having multiple meanings). With reference to characteristics of human beings, there are numerous abstractions of which intelligence, personality, authoritarian, and schizophrenia are but a few. For such terms, there is no single concrete designation.

There is a special category used in medicine and the behavioral sciences that relates to this abstract-concrete distinction, but is on the abstract side. The term is "construct." This term is found in scientific studies. It takes an expression and "constructs" a concrete definition based on it. That is, the scientist searches for possible observables or referents in the environment that are sufficient to render the word more denotatively exact and, importantly, are measurable. To be investigated scientifically, the term must be quantified or measured in some fashion (measurement refers to rules for the assignment of numbers in order to represent quantities of a variable in question). More simply, the scientist takes an abstract word and makes it more concrete and measurable [5].

Throughout the book, we will provide examples of patient complexity and related treatment modalities. At this point, we illustrate the process of making the abstract more concrete and understandable using the variables "intelligence" and "authoritarianism."

Intelligence

Let us now examine the process for constructing a measurable, concrete definition for the abstract term "intelligence" [1]. The initial step is to offer a tentative verbal definition. Intelligence is an aggregate or global capacity to act purposely, think rationally, and deal effectively with the environment [2]. The next step is termed "construct explication." This step involves concocting explicit concrete referents for the key components of the abstractions "act purposely," "think rationally," and "deal effectively with the environment." For example, traversing a maze from start to finish via a series of complicated pathways might be purposeful behavior; developing a sound deductive syllogism or evaluating whether the conclusion of a deductive argument is justified might exemplify rational thinking. Solving a problem necessary for survival might be an example of dealing effectively with the environment.

Now, in a simplified way, we have taken a word from common parlance, "intelligence," defined the term, and provided specific behaviors or referents for each component of the definition [3]. In so doing, the abstract word becomes more concrete or explicit. There are now referents that can be specified in the environment to "concretize" what hitherto was an abstract expression [4]. We can point to these concrete referents in a manner that facilitates communication [5]. Importantly, once numbers are assigned, the powerful tools of mathematics can be applied that include mathematical models and statistical analyses. One application following quantification is statistical evaluation using measuring instruments to determine "psychometric properties" that are important for evaluating the adequacy of a measuring instrument. Such properties are listed below:

Reliability

This term refers to several properties of a test or measurement procedure. It can refer to the consistency of measurement outcomes. If the instrument is administered twice, for example, within a 2-week time period, essentially the same results are obtained. This is called "test-retest" reliability. Conceptually, a test-retest "reliability coefficient" refers to the amount of measurement error in a test. If a test is 80% reliable, it has 20% error.

Another kind of reliability is "internal consistency." It is a statistic specifying the degree to which the test items are measuring information from the same domain of content. Do all items on a test about the solar system assess some aspect of the solar system? Does a test that purports to measure patient complexity have items that relate directly or indirectly to that subject matter? Cronbach's alpha coefficient is one often used statistic for evaluating internal consistency.

The standards for reliability differ according to whether the investigation is conducted within theoretical or applied research. The low standard for reliability is 0.70. When test results are used to make decisions about human beings, the standard is elevated to 0.80 and above.

Once a reliability coefficient has been computed, the standard error of measurement can be derived. If reliability is the extent to which an individual's test score is likely to maintain a consistent value with repeated administrations of the test, the standard error of measurement is the estimated distribution of those repeated test scores. And because of measurement error, those scores are not going to be identical. Again, if a test is 80% reliable, it has 20% measurement error. The standard error takes that 20% error estimate and indicates the discrepancy between average obtained scores on subsequent test administrations and the test-takers' "true" score, the score she/he would have achieved if the measure were perfectly reliable or error-free. The standard error of measurement yields a range within which the "true" score is probably found. Assuming a "normal" score distribution, a standard error of "2" and an obtained score of "50," it is 68% likely that the individual's true score is within the range of "48" to "52" [5].

Recall that a normal distribution is a probability distribution that is symmetrical or "bell shaped" in appearance. That is, most cases occur around the mean (the apex of the bell) with progressively declining frequencies of cases above and below the mean. Thus, in the United States, most individuals administered an IQ test will score about the mean of "100," whereas scores far above the mean (say "140") or far below the mean (say "20") occur at low frequencies or in the "tails" of the bell-shaped curve.

Inter-Judge Reliability

There are so-called "objective" tests in which anyone who scores the measurement instrument will get the same result. A familiar case in point is the multiple-choice classroom achievement test. For each four-alternative items, one alternative is deemed correct. Any person who judges the adequacy of a student's performance merely adds up the number of selected correct answers. There is essentially no error or unreliability of such measures due to scoring errors.

On "subjective" tests, performance is evaluated by ratings pertaining to verbal responses of the test-taker or judgments of observed behavior submitted by trained individuals. Here, a new source of error or unreliability pertains. Independent judges with access to the same observational data may yield different rating scores. Subjective measuring instruments of patient complexity, for example, include the VB ICM-CAG, previously discussed.

There are statistical procedures to ascertain the interrater reliability of subjective tests. All relate to the extent of agreement between or among independent judgments, the degree to which they assign the same score to the same rated variable. Like other reliability coefficients, they provide information about the amount of measurement error, and the likelihood that an obtained result can be replicated. And, like other forms of reliability, the 80% value is the low level of acceptability.

Reliability estimates for two judges can simply involve correlating their two ratings or comparing the average scores. A reasonable alternative is calculating the percentage of their overlapping scores (e.g., the number of agreement scores divided by the total number of scores). Because of the possibility of coincidental agreement, the "kappa" coefficient was concocted and involves the calculation of the percentage of agreement between or among judgments, corrected for chance (accidental or random agreement related to guessing) [6].

When there are more than two raters (the preferred condition), other reliability estimates are available. One is an adaptation of the kappa termed "Fleiss kappa"; the other main statistic of this type is the intraclass correlation [7]. This approach provides inferences regarding degree of similarity among rater means [8].

When disagreements are found between and among raters, investigations regarding verbal rating criteria are conducted. Perhaps instructions for judges are ambiguous or for other reasons misunderstood and need to be revised. Inexperienced raters may require further training that could involve discussions of disparities between their ratings and those of experienced "veterans."

Before proceeding to the topic of test validity, it is important to note that the value of the reliability coefficient places a limit on the degree to which a test is likely to be valid. In the extreme instance, the test has zero reliability. In that case the test could be replete with error. Logically, an instrument that only measures error cannot be valid. The amount of measurement error will be proportionate to the level of validity that can be achieved.

Validity

"Validity" refers to whether a test measures what it was designed for. Does a test that purports to measure political attitudes assess this construct? Often validity is evaluated with reference to some important criterion, for example, political attitudes and voting behavior, or intelligence and grade point average. Meller et al. [9] provide a pertinent example of the potential difficulty in applying these criteria to complex patients in their assessment of patients who displayed substance use problems and had both psychiatric and medical disorders.

Control

This term simply means the elimination of competing or alternative explanations for an outcome of interest. For instance, if the scientific hypothesis relates to whether a new medication for depressive disorder is actually effective, an investigator has to consider what other variables besides the new medication can reduce depressive symptoms. Hence, a primary consideration for control is a placebo group using an "active placebo," a pill that looks like actual medication but only produces an "active" tingling sensation without any ability to affect the biochemistry involved in depression. Participants are randomly assigned to the medication or placebo conditions and remain "blind" as to which group they are assigned. A pre-posttest of depression evaluates and compares changes in depression for the experimental and control groups. Nevertheless, even with the control, we are far from finished in the quest to eliminate competing explanations. Knowledge by medical personnel regarding which participants received the medication or placebo might influence their behavior toward the respective patients potentially influencing the results. We would therefore need to keep significant ancillary people, e.g., evaluators and parents associated with the study "blind" in this regard. We could expand to include other controls in this example, e.g., just the act of taking a pretest can influence scores on a posttest and would require another control group that just takes the two tests without medication or placebo.

Null Hypothesis

As mentioned, one generalization about the scientific method is that it is a set of techniques for reducing or expunging human error. However, consider the statement from Nobel laureate Richard Feynman, "the easiest person to fool is oneself," referring to "confirmatory bias" discussed earlier [10]. Scientists hope for a research result consistent with their theoretical notions. A common "non-biasing" approach to scientific research is therefore to search for the converse of their hoped-for outcome. This is the hypothesis that there will be no statistically significant findings from their research endeavor, the *null hypothesis*. The scientist attempts to disprove the positive hypothesis of theoretical interest. Then they allow the neutral, non-emotional techniques of mathematical statistics to decide the fate of the null versus alternative hypotheses.

Falsifiability

Related to the null hypothesis is the importance of falsifiability. This idea refers to whether the null hypothesis is testable. The null hypothesis is a statement of the potential for falsifiability. The example involving antidepressant medication can illustrate this principle. The null hypothesis states that there will be no statistical difference between the effects of an actual medication and a placebo on measured depression. Failure to find a significant statistical impact would provide a mathematical basis for acceptance of the null hypothesis, suggesting therefore that the (alternative) hypothesis of medication effectiveness has been tentatively falsified. Future replications of such a null finding would help to substantiate that claim (see below).

One novel way of thinking about falsifiability comes from Carl Sagan, an astronomer and astrophysicist [11]. He invites a visitor to meet a dragon who lives in Sagan's garage. They go into the garage and behold, there is no dragon. Sagan explains that the dragon is invisible. The visitor suggests putting flour on the garage floor such that the footprints could be observed. Sagan counters that the invisible dragon is suspended in the air. On and on, Sagan extricates the dragon from any hope of being encountered. There is no way to corroborate the existence of the dragon yet no way to reject or falsify the dragon's existence; it is outside the realm of science.

Replication

Finally, and perhaps surprisingly, there is no such thing as single well-controlled, rigorous investigation yielding a scientific "truth." A statistical rejection of the null hypothesis resulting in a probability that the finding has truth value is never absolute. Moreover, in any single study, there may be uncontrolled variables or other subtle errors of which the researcher was unaware. Hence, the importance of repeated investigations that converge and substantiate a scientific finding.

Important Statistical Methods

Research studies dealing with humans increasingly involve large numbers of participants utilizing several associated measures. The sight of data sets with thousands of participants and several test numbers associated with each name will, at first glance, seem overwhelming. Computer programs like SPSS are usually necessary for dealing with these situations.

Factor Analysis

Thankfully, there are statistical methods for reducing such data sets to render them manageable. The most familiar of these is called "factor analysis." The algorithms in factor analysis search copious amounts of data for patterns of covariation. Let us say that among administrated tests are a measure of vocabulary, verbal abstract reasoning, and one's general fund of knowledge. Factor analytic procedures indicate that persons who score high on vocabulary also have elevated scores on verbal abstract reasoning and general information. Correspondingly, individuals who score low on vocabulary have commensurate scores on the other two measures. The three tests can in effect be viewed as measuring the same thing, a category called "verbal comprehension." In this simple example, three separate measures associated with a collection of data are reduced to that single "factor." Scores on vocabulary, verbal abstract reasoning, and general knowledge are directly observed or "manifest variables." The common element of "verbal comprehension" remains unobserved until extracted through factor analysis. For this reason, a "factor" in the research literature is often referred to as a "latent" variable [12, 13].

ROC Curves

The acronym "ROC" refers to "receiver operating characteristics." This is a phrase from a technology developed during World War II for distinguishing radar signals that are accurate from those that were deemed "noise" or irrelevant. The technique, as currently employed in medicine and the behavioral sciences, is analogous to the original usage. ROC allows researchers and practitioners to use diagnostic test data to distinguish persons who have a disorder or a particular characteristic of interest (accurate detection) from those who do not. The term "curve" refers to a plot between "true positives" (e.g., those classified by the diagnostic test as having the disorder, confirmed, also called "sensitivity") and "false positives" (e.g., those classified by the diagnostic test as having the disorder, actually disconfirmed, also written "1-specificity", i.e. 1 minus specificity). From the curve, a score on the diagnostic test is derived that for subsequent test-takers maximizes true positives and minimizes false-positive rates [14].

Meta-Analysis

There are massive data sets that can be reduced via factor analysis. There are also large numbers of published studies on important topics in medicine and other disciplines that require integration. Do independent studies in the same given area yield identical or at least similar outcomes? Integrated literature reviews and literary summaries are the traditional approaches for answering this question. The "meta-analysis" is a technique involving an integration of independent investigations using the tools of mathematical statistics. Meta-analyses provide statistical data on study reliability and the degree of heterogeneity of results together with information about variables that may influence ("moderate") findings across studies. Axiomatically, these are attempts to summarize and integrate outcomes in a way that is more rigorous and inclusive than traditional literature reviews [15].

Multiple Correlation

The simple, two-variable correlation (also called "Pearson r" or "zero order") is the degree of relationship between two variables of interest. One familiar correlated relationship is between intelligence (the predictor variable) and grade point average ("GPA" the criterion variable). Based on an obtained correlation of this type, a high school freshman's score on an intelligence test can be used with fair accuracy to predict her or his GPA at the end of the academic year or even 4 years in the future. The use of a correlation coefficient in this way for prediction is termed "regression."

Obviously, intelligence is only one possible predictor, albeit an important one, of GPA. Other possible predictor variables might include achievement motivation and study skills. What if we combined all three predictor variables together in some fashion; could we then increase prediction accuracy? Indeed, potential predictors for GPA and numerous other criterion measures can be combined with resultant reduced errors of prediction. When two or more predictor variables are combined in relation to a single criterion variable, the statistical method is termed "multiple correlation," usually designated with a capital "R." Using the multiple R to predict is not surprisingly termed "multiple regression" [16].

Path Analysis (also see Chapters 46 and 47)

Path analysis is a subtype of multiple correlation in that the researcher is evaluating relationships between several independent variables and a single criterion measure. In contrast to multiple correlation, the goal in path analysis is to illuminate potential causal relationships.

You have been exposed to the oft-quoted aphorism, "correlation does not equal causation." This is an absolutely veridical statement. However, it is also true that a "causal" variable must be correlated with an "effect" variable. Correlation is a necessary aspect of causation. Cause and effect variables must be systematically related to one another. If a causal variable increases or decreases in strength, there must be an observable change in the "effect" variable.

A second necessary component in causation is that a causal variable must precede the effect variable. This is missing information when one deals solely with correlated data.

In a path analysis, existing knowledge of real-world time-ordering is incorporated in what is termed a "path model." As a simple example, a model of academic achievement would have study time as a preceding variable in the time-order with the assumption that study time is a causal variable of interest [17].

Path analysis attempts to simulate causation with the development of a "path model" in which hypothesized causal variables are presented as preceding the effect variable. The schematic representation goes from a left to right direction beginning with the presumed causal variables of interest. Moreover, there are two types of causation that are modeled: *direct* and *indirect*.

Direct and Indirect Effects in Path Analysis [18]

In the path diagram, a presumed direct effect is viewed as one that influences the dependent variable without being encumbered by other intervening factors. An indirect effect conversely is mediated by other variables in the path model. For example, Kamo et al. [19] investigated involvement is activities of daily living among older individuals (age 65 and above). The basic interest was in whether adequate nutrition levels affected involvement in daily activities. The results indicated nutrition had no direct effect but indirectly influenced performance of daily activities via improved general physical functioning. Turkoz et al. [18] investigated the effects of an antipsychotic medication (paliperidone) on depressive symptoms among persons with schizoaffective disorder. In the statistical analysis of the magnitude and significance of path variables, both direct and indirect effects were found. Specifically, paliperidone directly reduced depressed symptoms but also had an indirect impact via reducing both positive (e.g., auditory hallucinations) and negative (e.g., apathy) schizoaffective symptomatology.

The fundamental question addressed in path analysis is this: if the independent variables are causal in nature, what kinds of correlated results should be observed? After developing the path model, actual data are gathered and analyzed to ascertain the degree to which actual statistical relationships match those that were hypothesized.

Like the other statistical methods discussed, path analysis is not an approach a typical clinician can use with patients. Path analysis requires large numbers of participants and high-speed computer statistical programs. However, the principles of path analysis can be adapted for use with individual patients. This will be elaborated in a later chapter.

Structural Equation Modeling

The current clinical research literature is replete with references to "path analyses" and "structural equation modeling." Confusion exists regarding the similarities and differences between these approaches in relation to methodology and data analysis procedures. The simple fact is that if you examine a path diagram juxtaposed to structural equation schematics, you will be hard pressed to discern a difference. Indeed, and fundamentally, structural equation modeling is the same as path analysis specific to model development and statistical analyses. Both involve posited relationships between and among variables constituting a theoretical model. However, in structural equations, both manifest and latent variables (factors) are included in model formulation. This is the main difference between these two methods [20].

General Theoretical Modeling

"Modeling" involves formulating a "theory" from data or to be more precise creating a hypothesis regarding classification of patient variables and how they may interact. The basic procedures for model formulation are delineated below:

Moderation and Mediation: [21]

Any variable identified as having import in understanding patient complexity will be a part of a system of interrelationships. "Moderation" refers to a variable, usually a dichotomy, that changes a relationship within the system. Cognitive behavioral therapy is an independent variable that appears to reduce symptoms of depression in patients. That relationship may be changed via consideration of gender as a moderator. If the magnitude of the relationship is stronger for women in comparison to men, inserting gender into the system will result in a change; gender becomes a moderating variable in the system.

Example

In dealing with complex patients, let us say there is an observed strong relationship between the number and intensity of chronic conditions and measured pain levels. This is illustrated in Fig. 4.1.

We hypothesize that depressive disorder is a possible "mediator" of that relationship. We therefore correlate scores on a test for measuring depression with pain. We can then make a statement about the impact of depression on the magnitude of the chronic condition—pain. The possible outcomes are (a) no change; (b) partial mediation, i.e., depression and pain scores diminish the obtained relationship; and (c) full mediation, i.e., the relationship is 100%. Let us consider the last condition, full mediation. This case is compatible with the treatment of depressive disorder through both psychotherapy and antidepressant medication as treatments of choice for pain, and perhaps a reduced emphasis on other extant modalities, such as the use of pain medication. But before taking such a step, what

Fig. 4.1 Relationship (correlation) between chronic conditions (number and intensity) and the subjective experience of pain

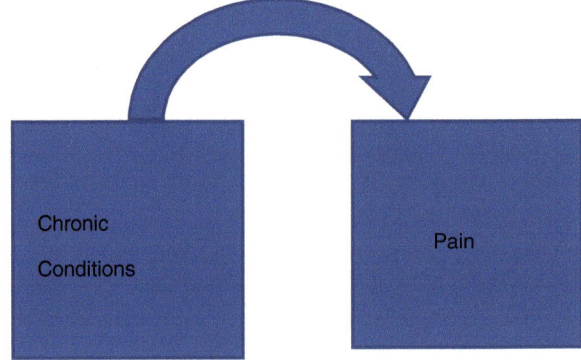

Chronic

Conditions

Pain

about possible moderating variables? Perhaps the effect of depressive disorder on pain levels only occurs with patients who are social isolates, without interpersonal supports. Or perhaps it only occurs with male patients, not female. Figure 4.2 illustrates depression as the mediating variable and social support or social isolation as moderating variables.

Assume that depressive disorder is a full mediator in Fig. 4.2. This would mean that the initial observed relationship between depressive disorder and pain was "absorbed" by depressive disorder, which in the illustration shows very strong correlations between both chronic conditions and pain. If we had simply and unquestionably accepted Fig. 4.1 correlation and not explored other nonobvious variables such as depressive disorder, the focus of treatment for pain may have missed the target.

However, we cannot stop there. Suppose the social dichotomy variable (support vs. isolation) was indeed a moderator and that only isolated patients with pain also display the mediating effect of depressive disorder. Now the presumed effective treatments for pain would be antidepressant medication and psychotherapy for isolated patients and perhaps a pain medication emphasis for patients with interpersonal supports.

What we have discussed in this section is a contemporary area of scientific methodology designed to deal with variables in complicated systems by formulating notions of variable relationships, hypothesized cause and effect, and variable interactions (mediation, moderation). Introduced earlier, this process is termed "structural equation modeling" and includes procedures for statistically testing the "fit" between a specified model and actual empirical data.

We are not suggesting that the typical clinician will have the capability or inclination for dealing with the large samples required to engage formally in the

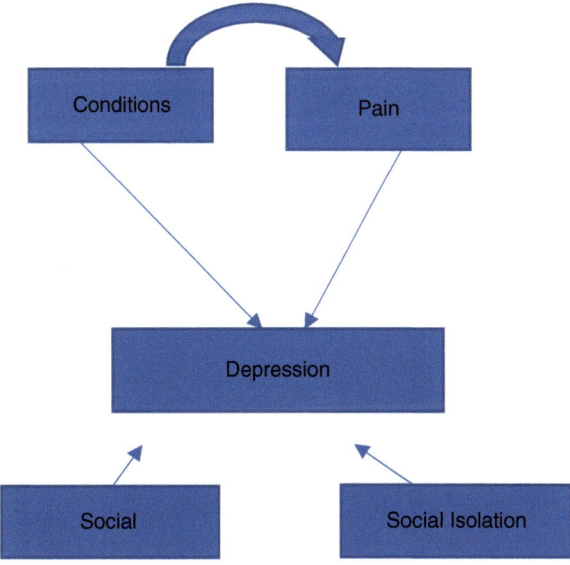

Fig. 4.2 Chronic conditions, pain relationship as mediated by depression and moderated by social support versus social isolation

process of structural equation modeling. However, tested and confirmed modifications of this model can be found increasingly in the literature, including models with import for clinicians working in small numbers with complex patients. Investigating such studies may help in finding the most efficient way of locating and dealing with "elusive variables."

We would also like to suggest that following the steps involved in "structural equation modeling" (path analysis) is a good way of conceptualizing and reasoning about complex clinical variables altogether. For example, constructing a clinical model informally (intuitively, loosely from data) and thinking about (diagramming) how the variables involved may moderate and mediate each other can be a useful activity for clarifying the nature and requirements of a complicated clinical situation.

In simplest terms, an independent variable is the causal or influential variable that impacts and effects the dependent variable. A moderating variable is a dichotomy, and refers to two comparison groups (e.g., male/female; passed/fail; religious/nonreligious; tall/short; high versus low socioeconomic status) that display significantly different degrees of magnitude on a correlated relationship. For example, the relationship between a specific treatment for a medical disorder and treatment outcomes may be moderated by socioeconomic differences. The treatment outcome relationship may be stronger and more positive for individuals with elevated socioeconomic standing who therefore have better support systems and access to medical professionals, and fewer economic stressors.

A mediating variable offers an explanation or reason why two other variables are correlated. For example, in a study on the effects of alcohol usage, a researcher finds a relationship between the amount of alcohol ingested and lung cancer and is perplexed as to why such a relationship should exist. Later, the investigator discovers that the participants in the study were also heavy tobacco smokers. Smoking was a mediating variable offering a cogent reason for the drinking-cancer relationship.

Moderation and Mediation: Any variable identified as having import in understanding patient complexity will be a part of a system of interrelationships. "Moderation" refers to a variable, usually a dichotomy, that changes a relationship within the system. Cognitive behavioral therapy is an independent variable that appears to reduce symptoms of depression in patients. That relationship may be changed via consideration of gender as a moderator. If the magnitude of the relationship is stronger for women in comparison to men, inserting gender into the system will result in a change; gender becomes a moderating variable in the system. As mentioned, a mediating variable is one that provides a potential explanation for an observed relationship (correlation).

The procedure for diagramming these situations is outlined below.

1. Select the dependent variable. What is the most salient variable? This will be the variable that patient and clinician view as the most important, the one that will be targeted for treatment. There may be more than one. If so, classify them in a hierarchical order of importance and select one.
2. Select the independent variable(s). This is the variable(s) that influence and cause changes in the dependent variable. First, the chosen independent variable(s)

supersedes and gives definition to the dependent variable(s). Second, if the strength of the independent variable(s) is increased or decreased, a change in the dependent variable will be observed. The relationship may be linear (most often the case), or nonlinear, positive, or inverse.

3. Moderating variable(s) and mediating variable(s). These are variable(s) that exist in between dependent and independent sets of variables and may influence their strength, direction, and character. There may be more than one of these types and sets of variables. For example, if the independent variable refers to an aptitude test score and the dependent variable is GPA, a measure of study skills is likely to be correlated with both variables and may provide an explanation for that relationship (see below).

We recommend that in concert with the clinician, the patient be enlisted to formulate a modeling sequence and construct a plausible diagram replete with rectangles and arrows. This diagram is meant to be a working model that can be changed as accumulating data dictate.

Turk and Meichenbaum [22] indicate that treatment is more likely to be effective if the patient perceives a connection between the nature of the presenting problem and treatment modality. As illustrated below, data from our patient shows a relationship between IQ and GPA. One reasonable treatment goal from the patient's perspective was to improve aptitude specifically by having a tutor work with her on areas of weakness: vocabulary and basic arithmetic. As illustrated, the clinician presented the diagram and explained that the aptitude-GPA relationship was strongly mediated by poor study skills. Moreover, the independent-dependent variable relationship was only mediated in this way for females. Therefore, the clinician suggested a specific behavioral program designed to improve efficacy of learning through modification of study habits. After this explanation, the patient understood the diagram and perceived the proposed behavioral program as appropriate for remediating her poor study skills. She also understood that while the model had credence, it needed to be further evaluated and that changing the model might be required.

Defining and classifying variables and how they interact in a system is the fundamental principle in theoretical modeling. Delineating the type of relationship, e.g., linear and curvilinear, adding the structural equations (types of correlation coefficients), and computing the degree of correspondence between the specified model and actual data requires large sample sizes and statistical knowledge. The issue is not unlike Einstein's "experiment in thought" that became the conceptual underpinnings for the theory of relativity. Recall that he was working as a patent clerk who had lulls in his workload, allotting him time to engage in one of his favorite pastime, ratiocinating (i.e., thinking).

The thought experiment that may have been engendered by watching construction workers in a building close by began with the mental image of a person falling through a great distance and Einstein's inference that this would negate gravitational pull during the acceleration of his or her body. Einstein reverted to the model of an individual within an unconstrained falling elevator to illustrate the point. This great experiment in thought was a foundation principle for the general theory of relativity. Einstein was certain of its validity, but he was not able to provide empirical substantiation. That task remained for others, most notably Arthur Stanley Eddington of Cambridge University during the solar eclipse of 1919.

In an analogous vein, we endorse the clinician engaging in thought experimentation where designated patient variables together with intuition and hypothesis formulations are used to create a theoretical model.

Summary

The scientific enterprise officially began in seventeenth-century England as an epistemological revolt against a prevailing notion that "truth" is the province of persons in authority and power. The procedures of the scientific method are designed to reduce error that may emanate not only from authoritarian edicts but also from human emotionality and biased reasoning. The data of science are therefore based on a neutral, bias-free tool-mathematical statistics. From a corpus of relevant scientific data, the clinician can then integrate other germane information gleaned in part from practitioner-client interactions and formulate a theoretical model of complex variable interactions.

References

1. Sprat T. History of the Royal Society of London. Knapton: Royal Society of London; 1734.
2. Chappell S-G. The Stanford encyclopedia of philosophy. In: Zalta N, editor.
3. Thurber S, Sheehan W, Roberts RJ. Attention deficit hyperactivity disorder and scientific epistemology. Dialog Philos Mental Neurosci. 2009;2:33–9.
4. Arnoult MD. Fundamentals of scientific method in psychology. Wm. 1972.
5. Nunnally JC, Bernstein I. Psychometric theory. 3rd ed. Maidenhead: McGraw Hill Higher Education; 1993.
6. McHugh ML. Interrater reliability: the kappa statistic. Biochem Med (Zagreb) [Internet]. 2012;22(3):276–82. https://doi.org/10.11613/bm.2012.031.
7. Landers R, Old Dominion University. Computing intraclass correlations (ICC) as estimates of interrater reliability in SPSS. The Winnower. Authorea, Inc.; 2015.
8. Koo TK, Li MY. A guideline of selecting and reporting intraclass correlation coefficients for reliability research. J Chiropr Med [Internet]. 2016;15(2):155–63. https://doi.org/10.1016/j.jcm.2016.02.012.
9. Meller W, Specker S, Schultz P, Kishi Y, Thurber S, Kathol R. Using the INTERMED complexity instrument for a retrospective analysis of patients presenting with medical illness, substance use disorder, and other psychiatric illnesses. Ann Clin Psychiatry. 2015;27(1):38–43.
10. Feynman R. The first principle is that you must not fool yourself. 1974.
11. Sagan C, Druyan A. The demon-haunted world: science as a candle in the dark. New York: Ballantine Books; 1997.
12. Fruchter B. Introduction to factor analysis. New York: Van Nostrand; 1954.
13. Rencher AC, Christensen WF. Methods of multivariate analysis: Rencher/methods. Hoboken, NJ: Wiley-Blackwell; 2012.

14. Zhou Y, Liu W, Zheng W, Wang C, Zhan Y, Lan X, et al. Predictors of response to repeated ketamine infusions in depression with suicidal ideation: an ROC curve analysis. J Affect Disord [Internet]. 2020;264:263–71.

15. Honts CR, Thurber S, Handler M. A comprehensive meta-analysis of the comparison question polygraph test. Appl Cogn Psychol [Internet]. 2021;35(2):411–27. https://doi.org/10.1002/acp.3779.

16. Kemp F. Applied multiple regression/correlation analysis for the behavioral sciences. J Royal Statistical Soc D [Internet]. 2003;52(4):691. https://doi.org/10.1046/jj.1467-9884.2003.t01-2-00383_4.x.

17. Fruchter B, Lasserre P. A comparison of path analysis and factor analysis for some simulated behavioral data. PsycEXTRA Dataset. APA; 1976.

18. Turkoz I, Fu D-J, Bossie CA, Alphs L. The direct and indirect effects of paliperidone extended-release on depressive symptoms in schizoaffective disorder: a path analysis. Innov Clin Neurosci. 2015;12(11–12):10–7.

19. Kamo T, Nishida Y. Direct and indirect effects of nutritional status, physical function and cognitive function on activities of daily living in Japanese older adults requiring long-term care: indirect effects of nutritional status. Geriatr Gerontol Int [Internet]. 2014;14(4):799–805. https://doi.org/10.1111/ggi.12169.

20. Shafiei M, Rezaei F, Sadeghi M. The role of childhood traumas, interpersonal problems, and contrast avoidance model in development of the generalized anxiety disorder: a structural equation modeling. Psychol Trauma [Internet]. 2022;14(3):377–85. https://doi.org/10.1037/tra0001117.

21. Giovazolias T, Paschalidi E. The effect of rejection sensitivity on fear of intimacy in emerging adulthood: a moderated-mediation model. Eur J Psychol Open [Internet]. 2022;81:1–12. https://doi.org/10.1024/2673-8627/a000019.

22. Pain B. Pain and behavioral medicine a cognitive-behavioral perspective. 1987.

Part IV

Nature vs Nurture and the Epigenome

[Part Introduction: In this part of the book, we touch on complexity introduced by the biochemical nature of human experience.

"Nature" refers to how genetics influence an individual's personality; "nurture" refers to the environment and how it impacts human development and behavior. Which has the bigger role is debated hotly in both philosophical and scientific circles. At stake here is not just cause but notably also cure. Traditional psychodynamic psychology (or "talk therapy") holds that remediation is largely a product of bidirectional or singularly directed human influence. Tell your biologically minded physician that you hold this truth to be self-evident and she may scoff at you. Say the opposite and she may approve. In the following chapters we begin to wrestle with the consequences of this dichotomy. Cure may be significantly dependent on which side prevails. Here is where the epigenome, the biochemistry behind individual traits and behavior, comes in.]

Nature-Nurture and the Epigenome

5

Introduction

Research on the epigenome provides a basis for denouement of the "nature versus nurture" debate. This resolution involves interactions among genetic and environmental determinants and is labeled "epigenetic dynamics." The epigenome, chemical compounds that switch on or deactivate genes, can be affected by factors in the environment, as well as the body's own chemistry (e.g., stressors). An epigenetic modification caused by nurture can in turn affect specific genetic functions with the potential for changing human physiology and behavior.

Perspectives on whether genetic predispositions or environmental influences dominate in determining human development and behavior have waxed and waned over the decades. In the extreme are the views of behaviorists John Watson and Sir Francis Galton. In one famous quotation, Watson stated: "Give me a dozen healthy infants and my own specified world to bring them up in and I'll guarantee to take any one at random and train him to become any type of specialist I might select." At the other extreme, Sir Francis Galton gave the world the concept of "eugenics," the ascendant power of heredity over environmental determinants [1].

The current perspective emphasizes that both nature and nurture conjointly contribute to the emergence and development of human characteristics in varying degrees, depending on the trait in question. It is exemplified by research being conducted at the Minnesota Center for Twin and Family Research at the University of Minnesota [2].

The epigenome represents the biochemistry through which environmental stimuli affect gene expression. In brief, this is the mechanism through which nurture influences nature. The influence of the epigenome explains why in adulthood two identical twins may differ in susceptibility to heart disease or the extent to which memory functions are maintained with age. Experiences in life will function to switch genes on or off, and those experiences occur differentially even in persons with identical genomes. Identical twins have cells with an identical DNA sequence but different patterns of gene expression. Enriching encounters, stress, exercise, sleep patterns, and drugs, among other influences, can all have an activating or deactivating impact on genes through epigenetic functions. It is important to note that for all of us, including monozygotic twins, the DNA nucleotide sequences are not changed, only the timing and expression of the genome.

The term "epigenome" was coined by Waddington in 1942 [3]. "Epi" connotes "something added." Yet, the activity of the epigenome is far beyond simple "addition." The epigenome is comprised of chemicals sending signals that communicate to the genome that its genes (strands of DNA) are to be turned on or off. Better put, "epi" is Greek for the English "above." It literally involves the formation of chemical "tags" that exist above and are attached to DNA molecules. Fundamentally, there are two main delineated epigenetic dynamics that will be discussed that can facilitate or impede "reading" the genetic code: transcription of the code into RNA and the eventual translation into body proteins.

Methylation [4]

One main type of epigenetic regulation involves direct effects on the DNA molecule. Specifically, the "chemical tags," methyl groups in this instance, are added to one of the nucleotide bases, usually involving C (cytosine) paired with G (guanine). This interaction produces methylcytosine, modifying the nucleotide and reducing the likelihood that the DNA molecule will be activated when this reaction occurs in the vicinity of the gene promoter.

This epigenetic dynamic is called "methylation." Following conception, each emerging cell has the same genetic material. It is the epigenetic chemical modification of methylation that provides some of the instruction and control in the embryo and fetus for cell differentiation and subsequent variegated tissue and organ development [4]. Note that methyl group is contained in commonly ingested foods such as eggs, cauliflower, peanuts, and wheat germ. This observation suggests that what we eat in our postnatal environment may affect DNA expression. Methylation also affects the degree to which DNA strands are "wound" around the histone. The tighter they are "spooled," the less likely gene actuation will occur.

Acetylation [5]

Acetylation is another chemical process that is a component of the epigenome. Acetylation "loosens" the DNA strand surrounding the histone core causing a "silenced" gene to be turned on. The operations subsumed by acetylation involve positively charged lysine amino acid molecules. When an acetyl group is transferred to the histones, there is a reduction of the lysine positive charge and an attendant diminution of DNA attraction to the histone, "loosening" the DNA molecule and increasing the likelihood of transcription.

There is vigorous research investigating other epigenetic processes that provide the "software" directing the "hardware" of the genome.

Noteworthy Environmental-Epigenome Interactions

As mentioned, one's epigenetic status can be affected by a variety of factors including lifestyle, types of nutrients ingested, and the nature of environmental encounters. Exemplars that pertain to medical and mental health professionals are briefly mentioned below:

Psychiatry and Psychology

The literature is replete with studies on the impact of adverse environmental exposures that influence epigenetic phenomena and in turn affect behavioral and emotional functioning. Below is a sampling of research in this domain.

Champagne and Mashoodh [6] reported on observations that methylation of the cortisol regulation genes in the developing fetus (assessed from fetal umbilical cord blood) relate to aversive emotional conditions experienced by the pregnant mothers. Postnatal follow-up indicated the children with the deactivated gene had difficulties dealing with stressful events 3 years in the future.

- Radtke et al. [7] investigated whether adverse events during childhood, including sexual, physical, and emotional abuse, subsequently affect the epigenome. A relationship was found between the number of such events and the methylation of genes associated with borderline personality disorder symptoms.
- Epigenetic research on schizophrenia implicates methylation of the reelin gene as a possible contributor to the disorder. Attenuation of the reelin protein in GABA-related neurons were hypothesized as disruptive to normal neuro-circuitry functions consistent with disorganized thinking in schizophrenia [8].
- Shimada et al. [9] reported a relationship between depression and methylated deactivation of genes involved in G-protein-coupled receptor signaling pathway, affecting a protein group involved both in the origin of depression and in the action of antidepressant medications.
- Finally, psychopharmacological treatments have been found to alter epigenetic regulatory mechanisms. For instance, valproic acid, used in the treatment of bipolar disorder, exerts influence via both histone acetylation and DNA methylation [10].

Medicine

Compared to other areas of medicine, cancer specialists appear to have an elevated interest in epigenetic phenomena [11]. Drugs that are DNA methylation inhibitors and drugs that affect histone acetylation exert a major influence on transcription in many plants and animals. One noteworthy study in this regard employed the drug temozolomide, a chemotherapeutic agent that destroys cancer cells in glioblastoma tumors through DNA methylation. In addition, the methylation process deactivates a gene that counteracts the effects of temozolomide [12].

- Dietary interventions based on known epigenetic components of Alzheimer's disease have been attempted with some reported success (e.g., cognitive improvements). The objective is silence possible causal genes pertinent to the disorder by increasing patient ingestions of methyl groups such as are found in vitamins B6 and B9 [13].
- Recent epigenetic research designed to improve failing vision has indicated favorable results. The study used mice as subjects but may have implications for declining vision in all mammals. Data from Harvard researchers indicated that reversing the effects of methylated genes (demethylation) can result in restored youthful DNA patterns yielding improvements in ganglion cells, promoting axon regeneration and improved vision in aging mice, with possible ramifications for treatment of human vision disorders [14].

Summary

In this chapter, we have added the epigenome to the patient complexity equation. We suggest that "nature versus nurture" is really a false dichotomy. Yes, genetic factors determine how the body works and may directly affect how humans behave. Yes, there are direct environment influences on behavior. But, moreover, as suggested in this brief chapter, nurture also affects nature and hence behavior more indirectly via promoting epigenetic regulation of gene expression.

References

1. Carey N. The epigenetics revolution: how modern biology is rewriting our understanding of genetics, disease, and inheritance. Tantor Audio; 2021.
2. William G Iacono MM. Minnesota center for twin and family research. www.cambridge.org.
3. Tronick E, Hunter RG. Waddington, dynamic systems, and epigenetics. Front Behav Neurosci. 2016;10:107.
4. Heijmans BT, Tobi EW, Lumey LH, Slagboom PE. The epigenome: archive of the prenatal environment. Epigenetics [Internet]. 2009;4(8):526–31. https://doi.org/10.4161/epi.4.8.10265.
5. Verdin E, Ott M. 50 years of protein acetylation: from gene regulation to epigenetics, metabolism and beyond. Nat Rev Mol Cell Biol [Internet]. 2015;16(4):258–64. https://doi.org/10.1038/nrm3931.
6. Champagne FA, Mashoodh R. Genes in context: gene–environment interplay and the origins of individual differences in behavior. Curr Dir Psychol Sci [Internet]. 2009;18(3):127–31. https://doi.org/10.1111/j.1467-8721.2009.01622.x.
7. Radtke KM, Schauer M, Gunter HM, Ruf-Leuschner M, Sill J, Meyer A, et al. Epigenetic modifications of the glucocorticoid receptor gene are associated with the vulnerability to psychopathology in childhood maltreatment. Transl Psychiatry [Internet]. 2015;5(5):e571. https://doi.org/10.1038/tp.2015.63.

8. Masterpasqua F. Psychology and epigenetics. Rev Gen Psychol [Internet]. 2009;13(3):194–201. https://doi.org/10.1037/a0016301.

9. Shimada M, Otowa T, Miyagawa T, Umekage T, Kawamura Y, Bundo M, et al. An epigenome-wide methylation study of healthy individuals with or without depressive symptoms. J Hum Genet [Internet]. 2018;63(3):319–26. https://doi.org/10.1038/s10038-017-0382-y.

10. Boks MPM. Epigenetic effects of currently used psychotropic drugs. In: Peedicayil J, Grayson DR, Avramopoulos D, editors. Epigenetics in psychiatry. Elsevier; 2014. p. 481–96.

11. Cheng Y, He C, Wang M, Ma X, Mo F, Yang S, et al. Targeting epigenetic regulators for cancer therapy: mechanisms and advances in clinical trials. Signal Transduct Target Ther [Internet]. 2019;4(1):62. https://doi.org/10.1038/s41392-019-0095-0.

12. Hegi ME, Diserens A-C, Gorlia T, Hamou M-F, de Tribolet N, Weller M, et al. MGMT gene silencing and benefit from temozolomide in glioblastoma. N Engl J Med [Internet]. 2005;352(10):997–1003. https://doi.org/10.1056/NEJMoa043331.

13. Chan TA, Glockner S, Yi JM, Chen W, Van Neste L, Cope L, et al. Convergence of mutation and epigenetic alterations identifies common genes in cancer that predict for poor prognosis. PLoS Med [Internet]. 2008;5(5):e114. https://doi.org/10.1371/journal.pmed.0050114.

14. Lu Y, Brommer B, Tian X, Krishnan A, Meer M, Wang C, et al. Reprogramming to recover youthful epigenetic information and restore vision. Nature [Internet]. 2020;588(7836):124–9. https://doi.org/10.1038/s41586-020-2975-4.

Awe

6

Introduction

The sense of awe is an emotional reaction to events characterized as "vast" or to experienced stimuli outside the domain of the usual and prototypical. A sense of "awe" is often described by scientists who peer through telescopes (immensity) or who observe the uniqueness and expansiveness of the microscopic world. A similar emotional reaction can occur with respect to the overwhelming experience of the clinician processing the complexity of intertwined variables experienced with a patient. When interpersonal awe occurs, it potentially opens the mind of the clinician to enhanced information gathering, cognitive processing, and empathic understanding.

Our clinical paradigm is centered on the essence of the therapeutic relationship. This relationship is the product of the collaborative experience of a patient working with medical or mental health professionals. We hold that the personal awareness of the impact of these interactions can be revelatory, at times analogous to a child's first encounter with a microscope or even of an astronomer's experience when contemplating the vastness of the universe they study. It is an experience that at times may defy comprehension.

We can only try to communicate the nature of this clinical experience through reference to the "awe" phenomenon. Awe is a powerful emotional response to overwhelming stimuli outside the realm of prototypic experiences. The awe experience can be engendered by interactions with humans and is not confined to experiences involving the physical world [1]. When "interpersonal awe" occurs in the context of the evaluation and treatment of a patient, there are several important cognitive changes that may occur for the medical/mental health professional.

49
S. A. Frankel et al., *Complexity in Health Care*,
https://doi.org/10.1007/978-3-031-14949-8_6

Piaget, Accommodation and Awe

The great Swiss psychologist Jean Piaget used a simple yet innovative procedure to investigate a type of cognitive adaptation he termed "accommodation." The test-taker, usually a child, is shown two tall, thin containers (A) and (B) half-filled with a green colored liquid. Both containers have identical levels of the liquid. The child is then allowed to examine two cylinders of the same size and shape. One of the cylinders is lightweight, made of aluminum. The other, again of the same size and shape, is made of lead and hence comparatively heavy. When the aluminum cylinder is placed in container (A), the level of the green liquid is raised about 1 inch. The child is then asked to predict the amount of displacement of the liquid in container (B) when the heavier lead cylinder is placed in that container. The child indicates a 3-inch increase and provides a rationale that the cylinder will take so much space "because it is heavier." The child made a prediction based on his/her developmental level of thinking. Now, Piaget places the lead cylinder into container (B). The child is observed to have a surprised expression as the liquid is displaced by only 1 inch, the same level produced by the aluminum cylinder in container (A). The test-taker is then asked for an explanation for the equality of the displacements [2].

The child in the above experiment arrived at the Piagetian laboratory with the idea or schema that liquid displacement is related to the weight of the solid object. That schema did not provide prediction accuracy. Now, the child needs to modify or "accommodate" its schema to account for the faulty prediction and to understand the displacement phenomenon observed (e.g., equivalent volume occupied by each cylinder).

When surprise bordering on awe occurs as with the child above, there is frequently an experience of disequilibrium. The subject's point of view, manner of thinking, and degree of understanding is challenged. The following cognitive features may take place:

1. Reduced attention to self-oriented concerns; awe makes the self seem small [3].
2. Awe then allows more attention to be available for attention to other-oriented concerns. It enhances theory of mind.
3. Awe is an epistemic emotion; it makes gaps in one's knowledge more apparent [4].
4. Awe may enhance fluency, flexibility, and creativity of thought [5].
5. Awe is the experience of being in the presence of something greater than oneself. It is an altered state of consciousness that can increase one's sense of connectedness to fellow beings [6].

Neuroscience and Awe (See Takano and Nomura [7])

It is also noteworthy that there is an emerging neuroscience basis for awe and the accompanying, generally expansive, cognitive changes. The cingulate gyrus (CG) plays a role in dealing with novel situations and in managing cognitive "shifts" and the accommodations necessary for understanding these [8]. The CG also mediates cognitive controls (e.g., detecting errors, monitoring conflicts in thought) necessary for understanding unique and novel events including attention and social emotions. CG connections with the middle temporal gyrus and supramarginal gyrus subserve self-other representations [7].

Physiology and Awe

The experience of awe has concomitant physiological effects in part associated with the autonomic nervous system. These effects may consist of stimulation from the sympathetic nervous system and calming effects at times mediated by the parasympathetic nervous system. The "diminished self" previously described and other cognitive changes mentioned may require a detachment from extraneous stimulation. There is a sense of humility, even calm, that is presumably engendered by parasympathetic stimulation, when one encounters phenomena such as the extraordinary vistas produced by the Hubble telescope, the Grand Canyon, and the world through a microscope, and we would aver when we contemplate the almost limitless internal worlds of patients with whom we work.

Interpersonal Awe

Although awe is usually engendered by overwhelming positive characteristics, it can also be evoked by stunning negative aspects of the physical world or personal attributes of fellow beings. The astrophysicist, for example, can be astonished with the expansion of the universe while simultaneously being apprehensive that the universe will expand until it ceases to exist. At times, interpersonal awe may also include astonishment and wonder based on horror about an individual. One of us (ST) has worked with persons who have performed remarkable antisocial acts. The vast complexity of interacting genetic and environmental variables that produced someone capable of exterminating 42 persons in 13 states was indeed astonishing (serial killer Thomas Eugene Creech) and engendered what might be termed a negative sense of awe.

We suggest that interpersonal awe often may be synonymous with the therapeutic bond that is the product of the paradigm shift we describe. The experience within this relationship can be as profound as seeing microbes when first looking through a microscope. By instigating an experience of interpersonal awe, a practitioner who facilitates a paradigm shift may activate fluency, flexibility, and creativity in the patient [9]. This characterization is not exaggerated. Try it out for yourself as part of a dedicated therapeutic relationship with a patient. A treater who is truly *involved* with his or her patient is likely to have an experience of discovery that defies and expands expectation. *Key to our proposed paradigm shift may be the uniqueness that results from bringing incongruent items (variables) together to guide the clinical work.*

Summary

A sense of awe has been discussed as a powerful emotional experience that may introduce a unique therapeutic component into the paradigm shift we describe. The clinical concomitants of awe often include reduced attention to oneself and enhanced attention and empathic concerns for others, including and perhaps most especially the patient. Added may be improved flexibility and creativity in delivery of therapeutic services.

References

1. Graziosi M, Yaden D. Interpersonal awe: exploring the social domain of awe elicitors. J Posit Psychol [Internet]. 2021;16(2):263–71. https://doi.org/10.1080/17439760.2019.1689422.
2. Phillips JL. The origins of intellect: Piaget's theory. San Francisco: Freeman; 1969.
3. Perlin JD, Li L. Why does awe have prosocial effects? New perspectives on awe and the small self. Perspect Psychol Sci [Internet]. 2020;15(2):291–308. https://doi.org/10.1177/1745691619886006.
4. McPhetres J. Oh, the things you don't know: awe promotes awareness of knowledge gaps and science interest. Cogn Emot [Internet]. 2019;33(8):1599–615. https://doi.org/10.108 0/02699931.2019.1585331.
5. Chirico A, Yaden DB. Awe: a self-transcendent and sometimes transformative emotion. In: The function of emotions. Cham: Springer; 2018. p. 221–33.
6. Yaden DB, Haidt J, Hood RW Jr, Vago DR, Newberg AB. The varieties of self-transcendent experience. Rev Gen Psychol [Internet]. 2017;21(2):143–60. https://doi.org/10.1037/gpr0000102.
7. Takano R, Nomura M. Neural representations of awe: distinguishing common and distinct neural mechanisms. Emotion [Internet]. 2020;22(4):669–77. https://doi.org/10.1037/emo0000771.
8. Guan F, Chen J, Chen O, Liu L, Zha Y. Awe and prosocial tendency. Curr Psychol [Internet]. 2019;38(4):1033–41. https://doi.org/10.1007/s12144-019-00244-7.
9. Chirico A, Cipresso P, Yaden DB, Biassoni F, Riva G, Gaggioli A. Effectiveness of immersive videos in inducing awe: an experimental study. Sci Rep [Internet]. 2017;7(1) https://doi.org/10.1038/s41598-017-01242-0.

Clinical Decision-Making

7

Daniel Kahneman and Decision-Making

Daniel Kahneman is a psychologist and Nobel laureate who made primary theoretical and research contributions to understanding the dynamics of decision-making. In his view, corroborated by other independent researchers, cognitive processes involved in making clinical decisions about human beings can be reduced to two fundamental systems [1–3]:

- **Type 1** is termed variously "intuitive," "automatic," "rapid," and "effortless." The clinician who processes information automatically follows what Edward Thorndike termed "the law of least effort." Higher-level cogitations and ratiocinations are readily retrieved without much effort. Information gathered about patients is interpreted via their own easily retrieved cognitive structures or "schema," which are overlearned and are "shortcuts" for making clinical inferences about patients. For experienced clinicians, these readily available intuitions can often be correct and accurate. However, without training and experience and use of the evaluative processes of the type 2 system, errors and biases can exist.
- **Type 2** processing is more effortful and analytic and involves deliberation. It may involve pondering research literature and considering specific guidelines or measurement procedures.

Both types of processing are necessary and important for accurate clinical judgments. If one type predominates, accuracy can be compromised. With training and experience, increased reliance on the type 1 approach is justified, especially when the clinician is aware of and guards against potential processing mistakes.

Some Potential Errors in Clinical Accuracy when Type 1 Processing Dominates [4]

Heuristics These are automatic, overlearned "shortcuts" for making inferences about patient characteristics. Perhaps the most important heuristic in type 1 processing is termed "representative." Here the clinician takes into short-term memory gathered information and impressions about the patient and compares this information to an existing mental representation of a "typical" patient in a particular diagnostic category. The rapid automatic type 1 processing with a representative heuristic may not yield an accurate conclusion. That is, the patient, especially one with complex interacting symptoms, may not "fit" a typical representation. In part, this book is geared toward the generation of the most accurate representative heuristics. Another area of heuristic concern as it relates to clinical judgment is the "affect heuristic" in which one's mood state or feelings about the patient influence clinical accuracy [5, 6].

Halo Effects These are cognitive biases that occur in either positive (positive halo) or negative directions (reverse halo effect). Halo effects relate to the sequence in which the clinician processes information. If the clinician's first impression is elevated and affirmative (the patient is in excellent physical health and appearance), this can influence later impressions (the mental health of the patient). In other words, the clinician may judge the patient to have better mental and emotional adjustment than is accurate because of a carryover from the initial impression. If that first impression is of a patient with physical problems and disheveled appearance, the reversed halo effect may transpire with adverse effects on judgment accuracy. The clinician's presuppositions about gender and race are subcategories with possible halo effect implications [7].

Attribution Errors An attribution is the assignment of causation for one's own behavior or the behaviors of others. Interestingly, there is a strong propensity to attribute our own behaviors to causes in the environment (external attribution), whereas when we observe the actions of others, the tendency is to explain behavior via a disposition or internal cause. Thus, a professor attributes poor academic achievement to low intelligence, while the underachieving student ascribes the problem to insipid instruction. With respect to clinical judgments, the clinician may erroneously assign a psychiatric diagnosis (internal, dispositional attribution) to a patient who in reality is having a reasonable reaction to a caustic environmental situation (i.e., the more accurate external attribution) [8].

Confirmation Bias Inaccurate inferences about patients from faulty heuristics, halo effects, and erroneous attributions can be maintained and indeed strengthened by the confirmation bias. Moreover, regardless of the other delineated errors we have discussed, this is one that can more generally pervade and adversely influence clinical judgments. It refers to a tendency to be attentive to and assimilate only information that conflates with our existing ideas or hypotheses about patients while correspondingly ignoring, distorting, and denying disconfirming information [9].

Formal Training for Improved Accuracy

A conscious-raising awareness of the errors and biases that can affect judgments is a first step in amelioration and accuracy improvement. More formally, two approaches have been found to be efficacious in promoting accuracy and can be integrated together.

Case-Based Learning (CBL) Exemplars and vignettes related to actual patients with varying degrees and patterns of complexity are typically presented to the student, culminating with each complex patient/case placed on a continuum of severity. The rationale for the level of severity is decided by the instructor. Ideally, students can interact with the instructor to achieve a satisfactory level of objectivity about the patient. Even without such dialogue, a presentation relatively free of biases and replete with explanations by a seasoned instructor can reach an acceptable level of accuracy. Vignettes facilitate the development of realistic, representative heuristics. Importantly, this is the approach used in this book. The book is replete with vignettes, relevant information about patients, and clinical data that are rationally integrated and discussed, with the objective of attaining as realistic a picture of the patient as possible [10, 11].

Cognitive Debiasing This method also uses vignettes each of which introduces a bias or fallacy with reminders to be aware of these (e.g., "don't forget the observer attributional error") and to counter the specific bias with neutrality, objectivity, and rationality. Although the vignettes presented in the text will not specifically focus on a potential errors and fallacies, the reader is encouraged to be cognizant of any thought intrusion they experience that perhaps constitute existing cognitive biases [12, 13].

Working Memory Working memory involves systems that construct and maintain processes that, in general, are critical for adaptation and adjustment. For mental health professionals, working memory consists of a limited amount of information that is active and facilitates the understanding and treatment of patients. Further, working memory includes a retrieval mechanism that searches for stored information that will aid in mutual problem-solving with patients. It also provides access to heuristics and factors that will impede accurate processing of information about patients such as cognitive biases. Hence, working memory includes the familiar "short-term memory" but also promotes "task-switching," the ability to switch back and forth from the immediate inputs from patients to germane stored information. Moreover, the brain structures and processes of working memory also maintain relevant information. More specifically, there are structures in the frontal cortex (e.g., left inferior frontal gyrus) and a subcortical structure (e.g., globus pallidus) that direct attention to the germane while filtering out the irrelevant.

Although less than perfect, working memory can thus facilitate attention to relevant facts and accurate processing of information about patients while providing access to stored information from one's professional training, formal education, and experiences with patients with the result of potentially reducing error in clinical judgments (related to the problems with heuristics, halo effects, attributional errors, and confirmation bias) [14, 15].

Summary

In this chapter, we have addressed the intuitive, effortless approach to information processing (Kahneman, type 1) in contrast to the more effortful, analytic procedure (Kahneman, type 2). The former is more likely to produce errors in decision-making, but both approaches can be important for producing accurate diagnoses and appropriate treatments. Specific cognitions that can lead to decision errors are presented. The case-based learning approach involves informational vignettes of actual patients and is considered a fundamental way for readers to acquire techniques for reducing biases and inaccuracies leading to improved precision of clinical judgments. Case-based learning will be the central element of this book and will involve actual patients with pronounced biopsychosocial complexities.

References

1. Kahneman D, Slovic P. Judgment under uncertainty: heuristics and biases. New York: Cambridge University Press; 1982.
2. Kahneman D, Kahneman D. Thinking, fast and slow. New York: Farrar, Straus and Giroux.
3. Kahneman D, Lovallo D, Sibony O. Before you make that big decision. Harv Bus Rev. 2011;89(6):50–60, 137.
4. Gilovich T, Kahneman GD. Heuristics and biases: the psychology of intuitive judgment. New York: Cambridge University Press; 2002.
5. Bowes SM, Ammirati RJ, Costello TH, Basterfield C, Lilienfeld SO. Cognitive biases, heuristics, and logical fallacies in clinical practice: a brief field guide for practicing clinicians and supervisors. Prof Psychol Res Pr [Internet]. 2020;51(5):435–45. https://doi.org/10.1037/pro0000309.
6. Talamas SN, Mavor KI, Perrett DI. Blinded by beauty: attractiveness bias and accurate perceptions of academic performance. PLoS One [Internet]. 2016;11(2):e0148284. https://doi.org/10.1371/journal.pone.0148284.
7. Nisbett RE, Wilson TD. The halo effect: evidence for unconscious alteration of judgments. J Pers Soc Psychol [Internet]. 1977;35(4):250–6. https://doi.org/10.1037//0022-3514.35.4.250.
8. Jones EE, Nisbett RE. The actor and the observer: divergent perceptions of the causes of behavior. Morristown, NJ: General Learning Press; 1971.
9. Nickerson RS. Confirmation bias: a ubiquitous phenomenon in many guises. Rev Gen Psychol. 1998;2(2):175–220.

10. Stark R, Kopp V, Fischer MR. Case-based learning with worked examples in complex domains: two experimental studies in undergraduate medical education. Learn Instr [Internet]. 2011;21(1):22–33. https://doi.org/10.1016/j.learninstruc.2009.10.001.

11. Nair SP, Shah T, Seth S, Pandit N, Shah GV. Case based learning: a method for better understanding of biochemistry in medical students. J Clin Diagn Res [Internet]. 2013;7(8):1576–8. https://doi.org/10.7860/JCDR/2013/5795.3212.

12. Croskerry P, Singhal G, Mamede S. Cognitive debiasing 1: origins of bias and theory of debiasing. BMJ Qual Saf [Internet]. 2013;22(Suppl 2):ii58–64. https://doi.org/10.1136/bmjqs-2012-001712.

13. Croskerry P, Singhal G, Mamede S. Cognitive debiasing 2: impediments to and strategies for change. BMJ Qual Saf [Internet]. 2013;22(Suppl 2):ii65–72. https://doi.org/10.1136/bmjqs-2012-001713.

14. Thurber S, Sheehan W, Roberts RJ. Viability of a compensatory working memory model of attention deficit hyperactivity disorder. Ir J Psychol [Internet]. 2011;32(3–4):144–57. https://doi.org/10.1080/03033910.2011.613191.

15. Baddeley A. Working memory, thought, and action. Oxford University Press; 2007.

Part V

Further Technical Considerations

[Part Introduction: In this part of the book, we depart from a linear, logic-based exposition and move to a mixed presentation constituted of both logic and clinical impression. Here we enter a world of seemingly infinite combinations of clinical details. Their singular or composite structures are all relevant to describing real-world clinical phenomenon. In the last part, we examined statistical rules for organizing these variables so they can be used to convey scientific meaning. In this part, we turn to the seeming disorganization of the real world of clinical events.]

Related Reading
Groves KS, Vance CM. Linear and nonlinear thinking: a multidimensional model and measure. J Creat Behav. 2015;49(2):111–36.

Introduction to Clinical Complexity

8

Introduction

A clinical situation involves myriad factors, including systemic medical disorders, comorbid psychiatric illness, sociocultural problems, and a range of other treatment-associated factors. Add that in clinical practice, there will be changes over time in the patient's personal life, as well as shifts in the patient's psychological and biological responses to treatment. It is when these types of factors are combined that the clinical situation moves from being straightforward (familiar to clinicians) to "complex."

As already noted, the structure of any clinical situation is remarkably complicated. It can be broken into components that can be named (e.g., personnel, treatment plan, the interactions occurring at any point between clinician and patient, the time frame for treatment, resources). Clinical events are also partially the product of the mind of the patient, the clinician, and the patient-clinician interacting. Further, little about any clinical situation is static. Pharmacological measures and epigenetic shifts regularly cause changes in the body's biochemical and genetic makeup. When summarized into discrete diagnostic categories clinical details tend to accrue or disappear. The resulting clinical configuration may (diagnostically) at points seem "solid" but is an abstraction and not necessarily true to experience for either patient or clinician.

These events are created both subjectively and intersubjectively. Further, little about any clinical situation is static (diseases evolve with or without treatment). There are shifts in the patient's treatment goals in response to emotion and external circumstances, e.g., death of a spouse, loss of a job. Pharmacological measures regularly cause shifts in the body's biochemical and genetic makeup (e.g., epigenetic shifts) some of which are transient, and some long-lasting or immutable. The core issue is not simply to name the influences, but to instead to arrange them in a useful way that reflects their clinical impact on the patient and treatment. Add factors

© The Author(s), under exclusive license to Springer Nature Switzerland AG 2023
S. A. Frankel et al., *Complexity in Health Care*,
https://doi.org/10.1007/978-3-031-14949-8_8

(variables) that combine with others to modify their clinical effect. When summarized by discrete diagnostic categories, clinical details tend to accrue or disappear. The resulting configuration may be descriptively coherent but is likely to be an abstraction that is not fully true to experience for either patient or practitioner.

Biological Complexity

Individual differences among human beings can basically be accounted for by genetic determinants shaped by environmental influences. The epigenome provides a conduit between the environment and the genome. Genetically, newborn infants will display differences in activity levels and responsiveness to environmental stimuli on the first day of life. Genetics and environmental interactions occur throughout the course of an individual's existence. Of interest, the strongest evidence for the direct influences of genes (termed "heritability," the percentage of a trait determined by genetic factors) have been reported for intelligence and the shyness-extroversion dimension.

For the practitioner, biological concerns encompass the individual's normal and malfunctioning physiology. Included are medical conditions. Biological complexity may, for example, involve genetic predispositions, traits with elevated heritability, and/or associated physical infirmities. Of heightened importance for the treating professional are the structures and functions of the human brain, for example, functions associated with the prefrontal cortex and/or deriving primarily from the normative or pathological roles of neurotransmitters.

Resolution

Working with all these variables as they affect the clinical situation is challenging and prioritizing them at times borders on the impossible. In ensuing chapters, we illustrate, by example, how this ranking may be accomplished. Which factors (variables) to emphasize clinically and at what points in treatment? Rating these in terms of importance to clinical outcome? Making a distinction between those factors that are of major clinical importance and those that are simply urgent to the patient because of personal suffering?

It would make sense for us to look for statistical ways of rating the importance and clinical urgency of each variable and the result of their interaction. But that sounds a lot easier than it is since in complex clinical situations, the numbers of interacting variables may be quite large and finding meaningful correlations between them based on their importance to outcome may not be easy. In the following chapters, we will further consider the nature of complex variables, what they are, and how to work with them.

Summary

After ascertaining the nature and patterns of a patient's complexity, the clinician must not be content with the notion that the arrived at diagnostic constellation is fixed and intransigent. She or he must be cognizant of and vigilant for shifts in the life and circumstances of that patient. Included are that person's reactions to changes in treatment and to extrinsic factors that are introduced in the course of the treatment process.

Our Clinical Model, The Place of Underrepresented Factors

9

Introduction

This chapter begins to expand the clinical situation by including clinical details that may seem inconsequential in a typical treatment. The illustrations present a range of medical, social, and personal determinants that when included in an illustration may actually emerge as central to either the patient, the practitioner, or both. Case descriptions are presented to illustrate different profiles of complexity. These profiles may indicate, for example, that in one instance, the prominent nature of the psychiatric illness may be the major expression of complexity, but with secondary and significant complicating problems related to ethnicity, economics, and access to treatment. Another case history may indicate that the dominant area of complexity resides in the disparity between the familiar nature of the systemic medical problems (diabetes mellitus) as perceived by the physician and the reality of the profound adjustment issues experienced by the patient related to diabetes management. Finally, patients with similar medical problems may have vastly different ancillary problems in other domains of complexity.

Clinical Illustration: Erin

The complexity of a representative clinical situation may be best illustrated by example. Erin's birth defects left her unable to bear children. Her parents did their best to hide these defects from physicians, skewing her diagnosis and treatments. She devolved into depression and then paranoia leaving her physicians grasping to understand what factors were primarily responsible for her dramatic clinical decline.

We are beginning to create a clinical model involving the non-exclusion of frequently discounted clinical variables such as the clinician's state of mind and/or

S. A. Frankel et al., *Complexity in Health Care*,
https://doi.org/10.1007/978-3-031-14949-8_9

of nonclinical but influential factors in the patient's life. Erin was born without a uterus and had only one kidney. This fact may have foreshadowed what was to come later. She worked assiduously in the family business, suddenly lapsed into psychosis at age 43, sued her parents for all their assets, and refused to be helped since she alleged that previously sympathetic family members had become her enemies. Other possible etiological issues included preexisting conflict with her irascible father, midlife onset of psychosis, and a new male partner hostile to her family. Her internist prescribed lorazepam. The result was a worsening of Erin's paranoia. No matter how attentive her internist and counselor became, nothing changed, at least until her anatomical defects and childlessness were recognized as central to her psychiatric deterioration.

Here is additional information about Erin. You already know about the surprising revelation about the congenital absence of Erin's uterus. Along with this abnormality, there was partial atresia of her vagina, a combination also known a Mullerian agenesis. It occurs in about 1 in 4500 female children [1].

As in Erin's case, these girls tend to present in mid to late adolescence (age 15–17) with amenorrhea. Twenty-five to 50% have urological problems including urinary irregularities. About 78% of affected women are hormonally normal with one or both ovaries intact. Penetrative sexual intercourse is not available to them without reconstructive surgery. As in Erin's case, external genitalia for the most part appear normal. The point is that there were lots of problems for Erin associated with her body. Just the thing for making a pubescent girl feel freakish and withdraw socially. The trauma associated with Erin's distorted physical maturation is now more comprehensible.

There is nothing remarkable about this example. Just a list of overlooked variables that might be contributing to the presenting medical and psychopathological situation. But here is the tricky part. To fully understand the patient, the importance and meaning (statistical weight) of each pertinent clinical variable needs to be determined and each needs to be carefully defined. The definitions must hold steady across time periods and clinical dimensions. Add the interaction of these variables with each other and the contribution of the patient's life situation, e.g., family disunity with interpersonal violence. The contribution of several independent clinical variables to the outcome, i.e., to the dependent variable, is operationalized in the statistical technique called multiple regression analysis. This operation is potentially relevant in complex cases like Erin's.

Ultimately, the following etiological factors proved salient in Erin's case. The patient's male partner, who lived in another country, was fueling her hostility toward her parents, she was using cocaine regularly, and on a visit to her physician, she had discovered that her single functioning kidney was failing. We will briefly discuss this case further. From this point, we will present case illustrations that like this one have contributions from more than one systemic medical, psychiatric, social, cultural, and interpersonal source.

The Problem of Simplification

Medical information and decisions by clinicians often rely on approximations (heuristic devices) because of the time, difficulty, expense, and sophistication required to collect and process quantities of information. For these reasons, clinicians are often compelled to leave out and/or conflate details. As already noted, clinical work emanates from multiple sources: patient, clinicians, and outside sources. Adding diverse perspectives: the patient's, the clinician's, and a public health perspective represents clinical work *as it is*. This amalgamation of contributing factors creates the basis for the complexity assessment and treatment approach we develop throughout this book. Dare to venture out into the field of clinical details and you will be in Mirkwood, a term used by Tolkien to describe a "legendary forest that ever moves," the "seventh piece of the staff of chaos" [2].

Tracking Variables

Of course, ferreting out the multifaceted complexity of the clinical situation may burden the clinician. How can a clinician think of all the contributing factors on the spur of the moment, the point at which many if not most clinical decisions are made? Our guess is that your response, as a reader, may be to wipe your brow and decide to return to "treatment as usual," reverting to comfortable algorithms.

Trying to describe this "field" of operation is reminiscent of quantum mechanics where location is inexact and the behavior of each quantum of mass-energy is only predictable within limits. There is a similar situation in medical diagnosis and treatment. Components of the clinical interaction are in constant flux, evolving in either a positive or negative direction. Apart from definable contributions, the thinking and sensibilities of each member of a treatment dyad or team interact and are ever shifting.

So, what does this situation foreshadow about clinical work? How can one predict treatment progress with any degree of certainty? In the following pages, we will approach this problem through case illustrations taking into consideration the result of the treatment partners having different mindsets, perspectives, backgrounds, and even goals.

Summary

Clinical complexity was illustrated with reference to the multiple symptom presentation of Erin. Included were variables that clinicians may habitually ignore or exclude from diagnostic formulations and/or treatment plans. Variables that are viewed as extraneous to the main targets of treatment are nonetheless often important for successful outcomes. In considering these underrepresented variables, reasoning processes like those used in the statistical operation called multiple regression analysis can be helpful.

References

1. Herlin M, Bjørn A-MB, Rasmussen M, Trolle B, Petersen MB. Prevalence and patient characteristics of Mayer–Rokitansky–Küster–Hauser syndrome: a nationwide registry-based study. Hum Reprod [Internet]. 2016;31(10):2384–90. https://doi.org/10.1093/humrep/dew220.
2. Tolkien JRR. The lord of the rings: fellowship of the ring. London: HarperCollins; 2003.

The Complexity of the Clinical "Field" Illustrated

10

Introduction

The complexity of clinical situations: a plethora of factors to consider. In this chapter, complexity is illustrated with four cases: a woman with chronic schizophrenia, a diabetic woman, and two men with heart disease. One's picture of a "clinically complex" situation in part boils down to the sectors of the clinical operation considered, and whose experience, the patient's or clinician's, is being observed. For example, the patient feels well taken care of, the patient's medical condition seems insolvable, the patient wants more support, side effects are in the foreground, and the case is uninteresting to the clinician. When the case is further broken into discrete diagnostic categories, details like these tend to disappear seeming to simplify the field of operation. The resulting picture is an abstraction, not necessarily true to experience for either patient or clinician. The following paragraphs are illustrative of the fine-grained complexity encountered in clinical work and provide examples that should aid in re-arriving at a realistic definition of "clinical complexity."

Clinical Illustration #1: A Woman with Chronic Schizophrenia, Complexity Based on Clinical Diagnosis (Jasmine)

Consider a patient who suffers from chronic schizophrenia that is in remission. She invariably belongs to one of several subtypes of schizophrenia. Her psychiatric illness is associated with social anxiety. Age, ethnicity, and economic capability count in determining her accessibility to treatment. Here are the facts. This patient

---

Three Clinical Illustrations: A Woman with Chronic Schizophrenia, a Diabetic Woman, and Two Men with Heart Disease.

S. A. Frankel et al., *Complexity in Health Care*,
https://doi.org/10.1007/978-3-031-14949-8_10

was born in Yemen, was university educated, and is 40 years of age. Her economic capability is restricted. We have hardly exhausted the details.

Components of the "clinical field" often include multiple participants that are both central and peripheral to the clinical operation (diagnosis and treatment of the disease(s)). Of these, the patient and the clinician are central. As in this case, the patient's family and cultural representatives (religious leaders, community) may be influential.

Sufficient? Not really. How does this patient understand her symptoms, in particular a delusion about an American plot to capture and kill her? Despite her anguish, she is admonished by her family to maintain the Muslim dress code by wearing a burka which partially blocks her vision and creates an appearance that distinguishes her from others.

Clinical Illustration #2: A Diabetic Patient (Beth), Complexity Introduced by Discrepancy Between Patient's and Clinician's Professional "Cultures"

You have a patient who has poorly controlled diabetes mellitus. Her vision is failing. She is developing a peripheral neuropathy with profound sensory loss in her left foot along with intermittent claudication due to impaired blood flow in both lower extremities. Is this a complex case?

Indeed, the patient's medical condition is troublesome and progressive. There is the potential loss of a toe and progressive sensory impairment. Certainly, her health situation is of serious concern to the patient but it is neither confusing nor obscure from a medical perspective. True, due its chronicity, its health effects are not fundamentally treatable and its progressive course is not likely to be reversed, at best only mitigated. From the physician's perspective, this is just another case of long-standing diabetes mellitus with typical complications.

On the other hand, to the patient, her medical problems are vexing. Involved is daily management of her insulin, at times tricky even with a calibrated insulin pump. With contemporary technology, nonetheless a patient with diabetes mellitus still needs to mind her diet, be prepared to spot infection, and remain cognizant of other diabetes mellitus-related complications.

Given that this case does not present a diagnostic challenge for a physician and the therapeutic challenge is familiar, where exactly is the complexity? Does clinical complexity exist mainly in the mind of the beholder (clinician or patient)? To a degree that seems to be true. A simple case for an internist, a tough haul for the patient. Facing patient and physician is the issue of recovery. How much of a struggle will managing the disease be for each participant? There are many factors that may influence our patient's recovery. For example, the duration of her disease, how well it has been managed to date, the patient's ongoing habits (nutrition, exercise, tobacco and alcohol use). Not to be missed is the patient's housing and financial circumstances. Altogether, this is only a partial list.

Clinical Illustration #3: Complexity with Patients Who Are Diagnostically Similar (Luke and Boris)

So, what personal and concrete (evidence-based) factors should go into the treatment strategy a physician creates? The details associated with this approach may seem picky or overcomplicating but look closely at two treatments involving a similar medical condition and demographics. Consider two 35-year-old men with coronary insufficiency, both Catholic and both from Brooklyn, New York, the coronary problems of both initially confirmed by EKG (electrocardiogram). It is no surprise that the pathology, the affected areas and functioning of the heart, may be different for each man. Since part of our objective is defining "clinical complexity," we need to look beneath the surface. Subject (a), Luke, is a physical trainer. He maintains an enviable exercise regimen. Subject (b), Boris, is undisciplined and uses alcohol almost every day. For both men, the cardiac illness by description is similar. However, prognosis based on habits could not be more dissimilar. Luke's father died at age 43 of a heart attack, while Boris' father lived to 95. This new information pulls for expansion of the criteria for defining clinical complexity and underscores the fallacy of a simple, static, diagnostic picture derived from limited clinical-demographic data.

Definition of Clinical Complexity, Continued

All in all, considering our case examples, a good candidate for a definition of "clinical complexity" turns out to be *the potential for overcoming blocks to health recovery in the context of a particular set of diagnoses and standard treatments* [1]. It would be logical but not always accurate to additionally subcategorize these complex patients according to personal circumstances such as housing and employment, while adding the place of comorbidity in limiting prospects for recovery. Balancing, however, for example, is the patient's physical and emotional resilience, the determination to master challenges including those that are medical. Any of these criteria would be helpful in describing the patient, none truly comprehensive.

Summary of Criteria Associated with Clinical Complexity

In summary, criteria that *may* be relevant for categorizing clinical complexity include:

- Structure of the case, i.e., number and type of clinically relevant case components such as comorbid diseases
- Numbers and types of clinicians involved

- Diagnoses
- Management challenges including the acuity and complexity of the clinical conditions at hand, e.g., schizophrenia and poorly controlled diabetes mellitus
- Goals of treatment, i.e., the achievement of expected or desired health and/or cost outcomes
- Context, i.e., the intersection of biological, psychological, social, and/or health system factors
- Level and quality of health care being received, e.g., a variety of "standard care"
- The patient's personal resilience, e.g., ability to manage disease and injury
- Other categories (such as those that distinguish Luke and Boris), e.g., genetic considerations

The component definitions above apply within the broad category of dysfunction and "disease." "Disease" can be defined as a medical or psychosocial dysfunction that adversely affects a person or group, impairing their ability to manage life within expectations. From a social perspective, dysfunction can result from a challenge to a person's or group's cultural norms. Dysfunction can be brought on or exacerbated in many ways including through economic hardship [2].

So far, the point we are attempting to illustrate is that the exclusion of seemingly inconsequential factors from clinical consideration is likely to introduce distortions into case formulation and treatment, for example:

- The family of the patient from Yemen, Jasmine, was hardly mentioned in our list of clinically relevant considerations (it is not strictly part of the medical picture) but may figure heavily in formulating the case management.
- Losing a toe may be traumatic for Beth, the second patient, since it is a stark reminder of things to come. Her physician may not appreciate the personal significance of this eventuality and its potential impact on her mood.
- Despite identical demographic factors, the prognosis for the two Brooklyn men is quite dissimilar, almost certainly reflecting stark differences in their self-management.

References

1. Kathol R, Andrew R, Squire M, Dehnel P. The integrated case management, manual: value-based assistance to complex medical and behavioral health patients. 2018.
2. Merriam-Webster Inc. Merriam Webster dictionary. Springfield, MO: Merriam Webster; 2004.

Formalizing the Clinical Field

11

Introduction

This chapter is focused on two case studies. In one, there are many extra-medical variables that read much like a mystery novel. There is a Machiavellian mother who threatens to exclude the patient, her son, from the family fortune. There are other intrafamilial relationship issues including those that primarily affect the patient's wife. His wife has recently had a liver transplant. She is hostile to the patient's mother-in-law and may be emotionally manipulating the patient. The second case involves a male Middle Eastern refugee worried about having contacted a disease before he left his country. He is affected by atrocities he witnessed there and is concerned about the well-being of the family he left behind. His ethnic affiliation may adversely influence his relationship with his Jewish physician. Both cases illustrate the challenge to the practitioner that may arise when dealing with the array of variables encountered during data collection.

Clinical observations are impressionistic. The depth and emotion incorporated in a clinical illustration is usually offered as a "real life" description of a patient, but it is not necessarily objectively "precise." Misrepresentation may be incorporated throughout the example. Here we discuss imprecise representations that can accompany collecting and reporting clinical data.

Clinical Illustrations: Seth and Mr. G.

S. A. Frankel et al., *Complexity in Health Care*,
https://doi.org/10.1007/978-3-031-14949-8_11

Clinical Illustration: Seth

Consider the case of Seth, a 49-year-old successful software developer. His personal life is on emergency footing since his 80-year-old mother, who manages this affluent family's finances with an "iron fist," has noticed that Seth's wife seems to be undermining the patient's mother's relationship with him. The more she thinks about this issue, the angrier she becomes, talking bitterly about "wanting to murder" Seth's wife and calling her such lovely names as "cunt." The mother's paranoia here is "crackling" but not provoked by Seth. In this example, several additional dimensions are added to the core clinical components of the treatment field. There are a wife, mother, siblings, and a family fortune at stake (consider the family money to be a significant clinically relevant variable since it heavily influences the clinical picture) with Seth's mother suddenly thinking of cutting Seth out of her will. Also added is that Seth's wife has just had a liver transplant for primary sclerosing cholangitis and may be holding Seth hostage through her suffering. Each new entry expands the complexity and gravity of the case, moving it beyond the "plain vanilla" of a single medical or socially based condition.

Seth's situation is certainly dynamic, dynamic because it is in motion and is the product of interacting psychological, social, and medical factors. Add subjectivity to the list. There is Seth's reality and the reality of those with whom he is interacting. Each person's "reality" is roughly separate. There are the joined experiences of each participant, different from each person's subjective experience individually. This state of mind is illustrated, for example, by the loyalty of Seth's siblings to their mother. Other factors at work include the actual challenge to the mother's titular position from her daughter-in-law.

Switch to Include Mr. G from Saudi Arabia

Mr. G. privately worries that he has carried a disease indigenous to the Middle East with him as he relocated to the United States. His dietary habits are restrictive and his anxiety after having previously witnessed ISIS-backed carnage is ever-present. He feels a need to protect his Middle Eastern family and is not fully transparent when questioned by medical personnel. He is cautious about medication, worrying that he could be victimized by a Jewish physician.

There actually is nothing unusual in either man's situation. In their essentials (incitements and responses), they are what you might find when you look up close at most any clinical situation. All physicians are trained to take a history that includes proximate and distant events. In addition to a medical history, they do a mental status assessment taking into consideration the patient's state of mind and chief complaints, including typical and atypical presentations. However, with the addition of clinical details, the situations may soon become overwhelming both conceptually and logistically. As a clinician in any clinical case, you have the choice of how completely to immerse yourself in clinical details. Notice that both of our cases become increasingly complicated as historical, clinical, and operational details are acknowledged.

Summarizing

Using Seth's case as an example of clinical complexity, there are multiple participants and a range of clinical issues to be managed:

- Seth's case is complicated by the presence of several ancillary "players" including his brother, sister, and others from his extended family who he assumes could be competitive for the wealth he could inherit.
- Seth and his mother are at loggerheads.
- Seth's wife's medical condition adds additional complexity to this mix.

Turning to Mr. G. These kinds of personal factors do not centrally figure in Mr. G.'s situation but are prominent in Seth's. They make Seth's clinical situation especially challenging. The challenges in Mr. G.'s case are more obscure and derive from his need to withhold and obscure clinically relevant facts.

OK, let's summarize. Our goal is to deconstruct complex clinical situations and in the process arrive at an increasingly satisfactory definition of clinical complexity. We have chosen clinically complex cases as our prototype clinical situations. Most include clinically complex patients with social (including family), cultural, and care delivery requirements.

Our specialized focus is on factors that are often discounted in clinical formulations and looked at by clinicians as details that are mainly distracting. How can we weight the clinical impact of Mr. G.'s worry about his health and his need to hide details from treating physicians? What about the impact of the distractions engineered by Seth's mother? These factors may not be included in typical diagnostic considerations. Omitting these clinical factors would create a false picture of each case and the requirements for its resolution.

Here is a partial list of these noncentral considerations as they presented in both cases.

For Mr. G

- A diagnosis that seemed to contradict the amphetamine-based treatment he received in Saudi Arabia.
- A history of trauma fostering distrust bordering on paranoia and instigating potential cultural clashes with clinicians.

For Seth

- Family discord fostered by a wife of whom his status-conscious mother disapproved.
- His wife's liver transplant.

Are these factors peripheral? Not in the least. To be added are physician-specific factors including cultural incongruity in Mr. G.'s case and inferred physician dislike of Seth's mother and her aristocratic ways.

Definition of Clinical Complexity Revisited

So, how does this information fit with our tentative understanding of clinical complexity as "the potential for progress toward health recovery in the context of a particular set of diagnoses and available treatments" (Kathol et al. 2018)? The phrase "particular set of diagnoses" could be replaced by "clinical challenges." After all, where do you fit cultural considerations or family disjunctions here? Neither are diagnoses per se. Both have typically been relegated to the periphery of diagnostic considerations. Instead, they are elements in a loose matrix of clinical influencers.

Part VI

Subjectivity and Intersubjectivity

[Part Introduction: How much of experience is verifiable? How much is a product of the mind in isolation? A major area in philosophy called hermeneutics is dedicated to this topic, the issue of interpretation. "Hermeneutics" is synonymous with "phenomenology" and "subjectivity." The abiding question is, what is real? What truly exists in the "real world" and what exists in the mind of another? Move to our patients and notice the extraordinary range of interpretations that can be attributed to their actions or intentions at any point and to their understanding of another. Attribution of meaning (interpretation) from one person to another is the sphere of subjectivity.]

Subjectivity

12

Introduction

In this chapter, we return to previously discussed cases, this time with a focus on "subjectivity." Subjectivity refers to the states of mind associated with emotions, opinions, and judgments. The topic of subjectivity includes variables that are often ignored or underestimated for their clinical importance. Included is both the patient's and clinician's subjectivity as well as their shared experience (intersubjectivity). Examples in this chapter include Seth's inner turmoil associated with separate conflicts with his mother and wife, as well as his fear of losing his inheritance. The extremely traumatic experiences of Mr. G., when in Saudi Arabia, are equally relevant.

The clinical field is typically represented as consisting of definable entities, for example, individual patients, family members, caregivers, and/or health-care systems. Supporting these "macroscopic factors" are a plethora of previously mentioned "microscopic" and hard-to-characterize factors (later discussed as "#3" variables). Included are those that are

- Biological, often subtly manifest in the clinical operation. Included are genetic and biochemical factors.
- Developmental, in part expressed as an individual's intellectual and physical capabilities.
- Personal, interpersonal, social, and cultural and health-care system.
- All of the above, in combination.

Clinical Illustrations: Seth and Mr. G. (2)

© The Author(s), under exclusive license to Springer Nature Switzerland AG 2023
S. A. Frankel et al., *Complexity in Health Care*,
https://doi.org/10.1007/978-3-031-14949-8_12

Subjectivity and Intersubjectivity: The Clinician's and Patient's States of Mind

As we move on, we will add the influence of new variables, the subjectivity and intersubjectivity of clinician, patient, and dyad on their judgments and decisions. Of note are clinically relevant factors associated with emotion, opinion, and "clinical judgment."

The segregation (what belongs in and out) of these factors is generally not carried out in a way that is entirely evidence-based. Inclusion and exclusion at least partially reflect the preferences of involved clinicians. Of particular interest to us are contributing items (variables) that are typically excluded or minimized in clinical descriptions. Categories excluded from our examples, but potentially quite relevant, include social, sociological-cultural, economic, and the ways these categories overlap and mix. We will also further elaborate on the influence of the subjectivity and intersubjectivity, e.g., Kahneman type 1 variables, of the clinician, patient, and dyad on their judgments and decisions.

The following illustrations give context to the clinical complexity items thus far elaborated.

Seth

When Seth, the previously mentioned 49-year-old software developer, came for treatment, his personal life was on emergency footing. His affluent mother alleged that Seth's wife was undermining her relationship with him. When considering Seth's anxiety, how should his being disenfranchised by his mother be included in the case formulation? What place to give to his wife's chronic illness? Is it the illness that most affects Seth or his wife's irritability? Seth's wife stubbornly insisted that Seth was flawed because he would not resist his mother's intrusion into their lives. Interestingly, when this case was discussed in a clinical conference, the wife's behavior and its effect on Seth were barely mentioned.

Hardly acknowledged is that subjective (e.g. non-quantifiable and non-verifiable) factors at times turn out to be the points of assumed greatest therapeutic impact. In Seth's case, being held hostage by his mother's vindictive behavior occupied him incessantly. His physician caught on that this might be the basis of Seth's chronic bewilderment and a variety of unrelenting physical symptoms. As the physician began to understand and address these concerns, Seth's medical symptoms including his "migraine" headaches began to mitigate.

And then how to determine which subjective factors have important clinical (personal) impact? Here's a statement by Harry Stack Sullivan citing the powerful affect subjective factors may have on treatment. "The child learns to focus his attention not only on behavior which brings approval but also on that which brings disapproval so as to avoid it" [1].

With this thought, we turn to research. But we are trapped there as well. No doubt there are clinical factors like the therapeutic relationship ("alliance") that have been well-studied and are credited as being central to patient compliance and change [2]. These factors are found in most successful treatments. But what are the independent variables that enhance the success of these treatments? How to differentiate them one from another and from other types of treatments? Sadly, we are, at least in part, forced back to intuition and clinical experience to see how clinical convictions arise and judge their clinical impact.

OK. So what? Do we not know what we are doing? Try the following examples of how the details of a patient's life can determine her or his focus can detract from the medical effort being made. It raises the question of how one can identify which issues are paramount to the patient, since these—in contrast to diagnostic designations—may determine how amenable the patient is to treatment.

We endeavor to be scientists and while a momentary retreat to principles derived from scientific research can be reassuring, there rarely is anything so plain about clinical work. It may look straightforward when formally discussed. However, clinical work is full of approximations and wrong calls (as well as correct ones) and is indeed influenced by subjectivity.

Mr. G.

Mr. G., as you know, had recently arrived from Saudi Arabia. He really did want to cooperate with his American physicians, but he had a secret he could not share for fear that the immigration authorities would trace and deport him. His hyperhidrosis had at one point almost cost him his life. Saudi Arabia in the summer is scorching. He and his family were in a sheltered place during a raid on their village. Mr. G. was hiding in a gutted car in unbearable heat. Finally, he lost consciousness. When he revived, he found himself in a primitive jail cell. He was arrested, and to identify him, he was tattooed. In the interim, over the ensuing 10 years, he had done his best to have the tattoos removed. But he couldn't fully complete the job. Mr. G. was petrified fearing that if the authorities, including his doctors, recognized that he had a "fugitive" background, he would be deported. Basing his treatment on what the American doctors knew simply did not lead to valid conclusions about correcting his excessive sweating and PTSD [3]. A fuller understanding of his history and its contribution to his current anxiety would be requisite to accurately understand and treat him.

Return to Seth

It would have been nice if Seth could get his mother off his mind. We then might have a neat clinical picture devoid of Seth's need to please his mother. However, Seth's almost fanatical loyalty was to his wife, and his wife was in mortal conflict with his mother. There was much more. (1) Seth could not easily let go of his inheritance. (2) While more implicit than overt, this objective, protecting his potential inheritance, relentlessly poisoned his relationship with his wife. (3) Complicating this situation further was Seth's paradoxical, private desire to repair the rift with his mother. In fact, bringing up the loss of that relationship frequently elicited tears from Seth. ("I do not understand it. My mother and I always were inseparable.") How do you categorize Seth's major conflicting sentiments (loyalty to mother, loyalty to wife, fear of losing his inheritance, desire to repair relationship with his mother) and the contribution of each to his current, complicated, clinical situation? Are any of these factors extraneous?

Summary

Subjectivity is defined, and the subjective elements of emotion, opinion, and clinical judgments are discussed. The first patient, Seth, had highly conflicted intrafamilial issues that included the potential loss of his inheritance. Mr. G., the second patient, had a history of major traumatic experiences and current concerns about his immigration status. The bilateral nature of subjectivity involving both patient and clinician is illustrated.

References

1. Sullivan HS. Conceptions of modern psychiatry. Ithaca, New York: Cornell University; 1945.
2. Barber JP, Muran JC. Alliance predicts patient outcome. New York: Guilford Publications; 2000.
3. Nemeroff CB, Bremner JD, Foa EB, Mayberg HS, North CS, Stein MB. Posttraumatic stress disorder: a state-of-the-science review. J Psychiatr Res. 2006;40(1):1–21. https://doi.org/10.1016/j.jpsychires.2005.07.005.

Further Reading: Subjectivity and Intersubjectivity in Clinical Work

Adkins V. Subjective Well-being: psychological predictors, social influences & economical aspects. Nova Science: Hauppauge, NY; 2015.
Atwood GE, Stolorow RD. Structures of subjectivity: explorations in psychoanalytic phenomenology and contextualism. 2nd ed. London, England: Routledge; 2014.

Gunnlaugson O, Scott C, Bai H, Sarath EW. The intersubjective turn: theoretical approaches to contemplative learning and inquiry across disciplines. Albany, NY: State University of New York Press; 2017.

Neisser J. The science of subjectivity. Basingstoke, England: Palgrave Macmillan; 2015.

Robbins R. Subjectivity, London. England: Red Globe Press; 2005.

Complexity in the Clinical Field, Revisited

13

Introduction

People can create their own clinical reality. Mark in this clinical example did just that by denying, to both others and himself, that he had an intractable disease. He created his own explanation for his medical condition and inappropriately concocted his own treatments.

A mysterious word, "complexity." It attracts and repels at the same time. As physicians, our subject matter is never simple. Just prick it with sharpened questions. Who exactly is the patient? Why is she or he here? What personal factors will encourage cooperation? Which will do the opposite?

Mark

Turning to our case. The patient, Mark, 37-years-old, had type 1 diabetes mellitus. This disease involves the malfunctioning of the endocrine system. He was not able to make enough insulin, meaning that he could not metabolize carbohydrates. The disease itself is often difficult to manage and is associated with myriad causal and exacerbating factors, many of which the typical diabetic patient may be unaware. Mark had a belief system concerning the causation and treatment of his diabetes. His ideas were at odds with evidence based medicine. His beliefs about cure focused on the remedial value of excessive, torturous physical exercise. Ironically, while intended for medical improvement, his personal remedies would undoubtedly have exacerbated his medical condition.

Clinical Illustration: Mark—Self-Created Complexity

S. A. Frankel et al., *Complexity in Health Care*,
https://doi.org/10.1007/978-3-031-14949-8_13

Simple! Or is it? This patient had antibodies that were destroying insulin-producing cells in his pancreas. The process had been insidious. It had apparently been present for a long time. As noted, he had type 1 diabetes mellitus. This type of diabetes can be further classified according to its cause as immune-mediated or idiopathic. It is responsible for approximately 10% of diabetes mellitus cases in North America and Europe. Most affected people are otherwise healthy and of a healthy weight before illness onset occurs.

Sensitivity and responsiveness to insulin are usually normal, especially in the early clinical stages. Type 1 diabetes mellitus can affect children or adults but was traditionally termed "juvenile diabetes" because most cases were first discovered in children. Type 1 diabetes mellitus can be accompanied by irregular and unpredictable blood glucose levels. Other complications include an impaired counter-regulatory response to low blood glucose, increased susceptibility to infection, gastroparesis (which leads to erratic absorption of dietary carbohydrates), and endocrinopathies (e.g., Addison's disease). These phenomena are believed to occur no more frequently than in 2% of persons with type 1 diabetes mellitus [1].

Why all this detail? Just so you know that this isn't simply an "a" leads to "b" situation." There are a variety of potential causes, exacerbating factors, and mediators. That means that there are many "a's" that could exacerbate or moderate the condition. But, oddly, it is also true that the person who has the diabetes is unlikely to be aware of most of these.

As you know, this situation is medically challenging enough. But, to our dismay as we think about treatment and adding a major personal complication was that the patient was an Olympic-level cyclist. He trained for 5 hours every day. Each time exerting himself to the point of excruciating pain.

But that is not all. In part what was behind this rigorous physical regimen was the patient's private belief that through laborious physical training, he could make his defective insulin-producing system work perfectly again. Here is how he saw it. "For each increment of exercise-induced pain I endure, new pancreatic cells, healthier ones, will be produced. It is as if my physical training funnels straight to my pancreas."

Note the additional category of complexity injected by Mark's idiosyncratic self-diagnosis. He had invented his own explanation for his disease. This explanation had evolved into a belief system. It is this view that became pervasive and countered his openness to accepting an evidence-based approach.

Of course, you as the medical observer are smarter than that. You cannot see any more connection between pancreatic repair and a rigorous fitness regimen than between uplifting thoughts and improved cognitive performance. We know that exercise is generally good for people, but how much and targeted for which areas of the body? What about sleep and nutrition, including dietary discipline? Our job at this point is to separate Mark's medical complexity into functional categories, categories that can accommodate evidence-based diagnostic and therapeutic procedures.

Let's summarize. There are a hierarchy of clinical considerations for this patient: current and potential symptoms (polydipsia, polyuria, retinopathy, peripheral neuropathy) and assumed biochemical derangement (pancreatic disability, loss of blood glucose control, possible immunological dysfunction). The progression of this disease is inevitably associated with biochemical and physiological derangement. Mismanagement of diabetes, at least at points, is likely to contribute, e.g., failure to monitor and adapt to glucose dysregulation.

So, where and how should we start our therapeutic intervention? How much emphasis should we give to each major and minor contributing factor? How do we incorporate our understanding of the patient's personal distortions and oversights?

Moving to an operationally useful definition of *clinical complexity*, what do we have? Should we, in part, base it on the number of medical professionals generally required to treat a case of this sort and/or the cost of medical resources required? How about the typicality/atypicality of the medical and social issues presented? How familiar are these to most physicians? Comorbidity may figure in heavily, each added disease and health domain in which treatment is carried out creating additional technical and logistical challenges.

Since you, as the reader, probably are a physician or an allied health professional, it should not be hard to imagine yourself treating this patient. We started with type 1 diabetes mellitus, a familiar clinical entity. We then added the patient's anxieties and rigorous physical regimen to the picture. Ordinarily, regular exercise is highly desirable for diabetics. This patient, however, exercised with a vengeance and at the same time was a bit sloppy about monitoring his blood glucose. Complicating his physical stress was his peculiar habit of going to bed at 2:00 A.M., in part because he did "his best work" at late hours. Also, while usually a reasonable person, he was tenacious about guarding his "habits."

Incidentally, it occurs to us that most clinicians are constantly faced with this level of complexity, but for practical reasons, and, yes, often to preserve their sanity, they may not be inclined to dive into the kind of treacherous personal waters introduced by this man's habits, including his devotion to punishing physical training.

The management challenge of this situation is evident. The situation itself is not medically complex. However, *managing* it is. Mark had invented his own explanation for his disease and his own ideas about treatment. He had no understanding of the emotional basis of his behavior, i.e., conviction that his diabetes could get worse and even kill him unless he subjected himself to strenuous physical training.

On exploration, it turns out that Mark's father died at age 36 from a brain hemorrhage (when Mark was 12). His father's death had haunted Mark ever since. It was not fundamentally Mark's diabetes that frightened him and formed the basis of his obsession with physical exceptionalism. The diabetes appears to have primarily served as a vehicle for focusing Mark's anxiety. Basically, it may have been the sudden and unforgiving impact, the traumatic effect of his father's untimely death linked to his own fear of death that explains Mark's idiosyncratic management of his own clinical situation.

Here we have a new addition to our repertoire of factors potentially associated with clinical complexity. Contributions may come from the patient's present, past, or imagination. At times, as in the case of our schizophrenic woman, "imagination" may contribute and can in the extreme be manifest as a delusion. These factors impact treatment and may affect patient progress. Clinical complexity expands as we endeavor to discover dimensions that are neither overt nor suspected. At this point, we are challenged to discover ways to unpack these complexity factors as well as gauge the extent of their impact.

Summary

Mark had elevated the overall clinical complexity of his disorder with his borderline delusional beliefs about his illness. In turn, his belief system engendered behaviors (e.g., torturous, excessive physical exercise) that were at odds with evidence-based treatment for his disease.

Reference

1. Allman T. Diabetes (genes & disease). New York: Chelsea House; 2008.

Part VII

Working with Clinical Complexity, the Empirical-Collaborative Method

[Part Introduction: Sorting out complex clinical data requires both deductive and inductive reasoning. The empirical-collaborative (EC) method involves the collection of empirical (observable) data, followed by a rational analysis and integration of those data, hypothesis formulations, and treatment planning with a primary focus on cooperative patient-clinician interactions throughout this process.

There are a number of associated professionals that may be involved in this process, including a case manager trained in nursing or social work, or physician assistants. Because of the complexity of clinical situations, and the scarcity and expense of physician's time these ancillary personnel are both essential and ubiquitous in the medical care system.]

Information Gathering and Integration

14

Introduction

Data gathering: While much clinical data comes from informal exchanges between clinician and patient, the empirical-collaborative (E-C) procedure can also be used with formal clinical assessments to ferret out hidden or obscure clinical information. Several examples are given below.

The work of the practitioner begins with data collection. Amassing data is the first step in the "empirical-collaborative method" (also see Chapter 10 of this book). In this chapter, formal interview protocols (e.g., diagnostic interviews, validated psychometric inventories) are detailed and followed by a discussion of clinical reasoning, e.g., inductive or deductive, appropriate for the processing of the gathered data. Emphasis in this chapter is on a generally unfamiliar subtype of inductive reasoning termed "abduction."

This chapter begins with exploration of our method for working with and gaining information from complex clinical data using the empirical-collaborative (E-C) method. While much clinical data comes from informal exchanges between clinician and patient, the empirical-collaborative (E-C) procedure can also be used adjunctively with formal clinical assessments. Several of these are discussed below. The collected data are then integrated by the clinician who, together with the patient, formulates diagnostic and best-treatment hypotheses.

Diagnostic Interview

Answers to diagnostic questions, such as those below, can provide clues to variables that may be central to the presenting problem. Examples of common questions found in psychometric assessment protocols include: Why are you here today?

What kind of a person are you? How would you describe yourself? If you could change one thing about yourself or your condition, what would that be? and what would you like to be able to do in 1 year that you are not doing now?

Functional Analysis

This category refers to an investigation of the environmental context in which an identified variable tends to occur with respect to antecedent conditions, consequences, frequency, and intensity of the identified variable. Self-report questionnaires and rating scales completed by significant others are typical assessment methods used. It could be found that aggression occurs with more frequency and intensity in the job setting than in the home and that a frustrating event is the typical precursor to the appearance of this aggression. A *functional analysis* will also suggest whether the outcome is important in maintaining symptomatology. Verbal aggression in the workplace may facilitate avoidance of persons who are disliked, for example.

Self-Monitoring

The patient is asked to keep track of the identified variable and associated thoughts. For instance, she or he records a number at the end of each waking hour representing the degree of depression. In addition, the patient writes down the main topic of thought that occurred during the hour.

Inventories

There are a variety of often lengthy psychological inventories designed to measure variables that may have relevance for treatment. The Minnesota Multiphasic Personality Inventory-2 (MMPI-2) is perhaps most often used in this regard. In the original construction of the instrument, persons with known psychiatric disorders answered 500 or so questions responding true or false [1]. If a subsequent test-taker answers the items like persons with bipolar disorder, this response allows a tentative inference that a manic episode could be a variable of interest. These inventories also have "validity" subscales that check for responses that are deliberately falsified. The current MMPI-2 consists of 567 items with multiple scales and subscales including validity scales.

Standardized Quantification of Specific Variables

There are several psychometric scales that purport to assess specific aspects of validity. Self-report and rating scales specific to symptoms of emotional dysfunctions, risk of self-injury, cognitive impairment, aggression, and the whole gamut of DSM-5 diagnostic criteria are available. Obviously, the clinician should choose a measurement instrument with due regard to its demonstrated validity and reliability, sensitivity, specificity, and appropriateness for the patient. Of particular importance for this book are instruments designed to measure patient complexity and provide operational definitions for its evaluation. However, such measures have apparently not yet proven reliable and feasible enough for practitioners to adopt them for regular use.

Reference

1. Butcher JN, Williams CL. Personality assessment with the MMPI-2: historical roots, international adaptations, and current challenges. Appl Psychol Health Well Being. 2009;1(1):105–35. https://doi.org/10.1111/j.1758-0854.2008.01007.x.

Clinical Reasoning

15

Introduction

Types of clinical reasoning are explicated and discussed in this chapter. Not all logical systems rely on formal rules. For our work, we find ourselves particularly interested in a system of logic called "abductive" reasoning. It, like Bayes' statistics, encourages creative thinking by allowing for extrapolation using previously obtained data.

Clinical data are analyzed by the clinician and integrated via logical reasoning and hypothesis formulations related to possible causal variables, and variables, that may moderate or mediate relationships between and among variables.

Logical Analyses

The empirical-collaborative (E-C) approach involves a familiar type of logical-clinical reasoning, termed *induction*, deriving general conclusions from specific items of information. In contrast, deductive reasoning, from general to specific (e.g., the well-known Aristotelian syllogism), is characteristic of controlled, scientific investigations and is often termed "hypothetico-deductive." The investigator formulates a general hypothesis and gathers subsequent data to confirm or deny the hypothetical formulation. This type of reasoning is the basis for experimental clinical research but is not explicitly a part of the empirical-collaborative method.

The rational work of the clinician is by necessity *inductive* because the nature of the presenting and accumulating data requires this type of reasoning. The patient presents specific data about personally problematic experiences. Inductive thinking is mandated to conceptualize these experiences and the integration with other facets of patient experience follows.

General inductive reasoning, however, can be juxtaposed and enlarged by a special subtype of reasoning termed "abduction." Abductive reasoning is not demanded by the nature of the presented clinical information. But it is an essential part of the paradigm shift we have developed; indeed, it is essential to E-C interactions.

Abductive Reasoning

As we proceeded through case studies and patient anecdotes, we could identify an amalgamation of inductive and deductive reasoning in processing clinical data and eventually when formulating treatment interventions. But there seemed to be a missing cognitive element that is rarely, if ever, discussed in clinical literature based on familiar logical operations. It is termed "abduction." The term goes beyond induction and deduction to describe the cognitive activities that comprise an important aspect of our "revised paradigm shift." This principle is illustrated in SAF's interaction with Michael (a case to be discussed later in Chap. 48). Here there were two steps of discovery: (1) SAF's recognition of how his desire for a new patient was confounding his clinical judgment and (2) uncovering Michael's legal problems.

Abduction goes further than obtaining general and specific logical conclusions. Abduction seeks explanations beyond logic. The clinician listens to the utterances of a patient and integrates word meanings and word referents with other gathered data. The clinician abductively decodes information and concocts potential explanations for the words of the patient that fit with aggregated clinical findings. This rational processing results in what the clinician considers the best explanation for the information at hand. However, other explanations remain as viable until and unless eliminated by subsequent data. The clinician using abductive reasoning always maintains an openness to changing explanations and an intention to expunge unsatisfactory conclusions as accumulating data dictate [1].

The Clinical Value of the E-C Method

Think of the experience of working inductively both as the clinician and as the patient. You take a clinical moment like the one involving a patient's lack of civility. You pick at it, exhaustively questioning the patient, unpacking details about that person's experience with their disease and treatment. The process may be intense, the patient experiencing flickerings of understanding as the confrontation with the patient's problems is orchestrated. It is not just the patient who may be influenced in this evolving process. It is the clinician as well. And even if you focus attention diagnostically and therapeutically on the patient's angry demeanor, you must keep in mind that this single issue is embedded with several, perhaps many, other important clinical variables that cannot be ignored.

Goal of the E-C Method

The product of the cohesion being described is improved ability to make an accurate clinical assessment. At each step in the empirical-collaborative process, the patient and clinician come closer to understanding the clinical situation with accuracy (as judged by their ability to predict clinical developments) and to comprehend the needs, limitations, and strengths of the patient. In summary, the E-C method is not just useful diagnostically but also in helping the patient to feel "heard" and understood.

In concert with the patient's input, the clinician can now formulate a type of "causal path diagram" (see Chapters 46–47) that incorporates the variables that are most urgently in need of acknowledgment and amelioration. Added are intervention methods and projections about what is required for successful treatment. Finally, there are judgments about how variables interact. The clinician integrates what is known about the patient from the empirical-collaborative procedures combined with intuitions. Educated hypotheses and conjectures are integrated via abductive reasoning.

Summary

Assessment methods that include diagnostic interviews, functional analysis, self-monitoring, personality inventories, self-reports, and rating scales have been mentioned. In concert with information gleaned from patient-treater interactions, the assessment findings are processed by the clinician as part of the empirical-collaborative approach. Emphasis is placed on abductive reasoning, formulating hypotheses based upon accumulating data as well as what measures will be meaningful to the patient. Abductive logic is collaborative in nature. Hypotheses are modified to be consistent with changes in data and in patient understanding and acceptance. This process is foundational to the empirical-collaborative perspective.

Reference

1. Åsvoll H. Abduction, deduction and induction: can these concepts be used for an understanding of methodological processes in interpretative case studies? Int J Qualit Stud Edu. 2013;27(3):289–307.

Further Reading

Lee PM. Bayesian Statistics: An Introduction (3rd ed.). Hodder Arnold; 2004.

Reasoning (Logic) Used in Clinical Work

Altable S. The logical structure of clinical judgment and its relation to medical and psychiatric semiology. Psychopathology. 2012;45(6):344–51.

van Baalen S, Boon M, Verhoef P. From clinical decision support to clinical reasoning support systems. J Eval Clin Pract. 2021;27(3):520–8.

Brown T, Shah S. Evidence-based clinical reasoning in medicine. PMPHj: Shelton, CT; 2012.

Barro S, Marin R. Fuzzy logic in medicine. Heidelberg, Germany: Physica-Verlag; 2010.

Part VIII

Creating and Maintaining a Therapeutic Relationship

[Part Introduction: In this part of the book, we describe clinical work that emphasizes surprise and disjunction for the purpose of facilitating clinical progress. The clinician assists in the creation and recognition of novel therapeutic/clinical moments. Focusing on these events replicates principles of interpersonal psychotherapy. However, added is the element of disjunction leading to creativity, new ways of thinking about clinical change and how it occurs.]

Failure to Form a Collaborative Relationship with the Patient

16

Introduction

Much of clinical psychiatry is structured according to heuristics, fixed categories (e.g., diagnoses) and formulas that specify how they work together. To be maximally effective, a clinician needs to be guided by experience and clinical intuition as much as by algorithm and formal procedure. The clinician must "feel" the patient and believe he or she understands (intuitively and by interview) what that person wants and needs from treatment and with what priority. Our goal is to find better, targeted ways to describe and manage these complex clinical situations.

Ethical and procedural rules governing treatment often undermine clinician intuition. Clinicians, for example, are often guided by rules that limit self-disclosure and ensure that the patient will have limited information about the clinician. Adhering to these guidelines may alienate the patient, even render the treating person threatening. The best clinicians know this intuitively and can methodically negotiate interpersonally difficult clinical situations with minimal practitioner obstruction to treatment.

Dynamic Features of Treatment

Treatment conducted according to formula also minimizes the fact that change is inherent in all treatment; improvement or decline in the patient's medical and emotional status is inevitable in treatment. Treatment parameters often need to be adjusted accordingly. The same applies to the patient's environment. It is rarely static. In fact, the circumstances of a patient's life may shift, often radically, during treatment.

Clinical Illustration: Herb—A Patient with Secrets

In summary, most clinical situations do not fully conform to any standard model for how the contributing parts interact and how they may conspire to mitigate or recreate the patient's distress and/or maintain or exacerbate that person's medical-personal difficulties.

Clinical Illustration: Herb—Polyarteritis Nodosa (PAN)[1]

In the following clinical illustration, one author, SAF, discusses processes involved in the initiation and maintenance of a productive treatment relationship. The initial contact sets a frame. A relationship is then built incrementally. In this case study a collaborative relationship was not achieved. A core part of the problem was the patient's unwillingness to disclose his consternation about his increasingly debilitating medical disorder to his wife, himself, and even his physician.

Herb is a 45-year-old CEO of a computer supply company and a father of two. His knees are painful when he walks. He is sure nothing serious is wrong with him. Oh, but he did notice blood in the toilet after a bowel movement last week. Truthfully, he would like to pay more attention to his health but says he "cannot possibly" take time away from work since a new and in ways more advanced computer supply company (competing with his company) has moved to his geographical area. Privately, he worries that because of the anticipated time crunch from health concerns, he will have to give up activities he considers indispensable to his well-being, like competitive running.

By the way, his sex life is also suffering, but that is his secret. Honestly, he admits, he may have lost interest in sex but his wife has not. He feels humiliated about that observation.

Herb becomes impassioned as he talks. Keeping up a "front" not just for others including his wife but also for himself has been stressful. He really does not want to admit he is failing—his knees, his immune system, and his waning interest in sex.

Most clinical situations involve specific variables subtracting from or reinforcing each other. In addition, these clinical items fluctuate in their influence over time.

---

[1] Polyarteritis nodosa (PAN) is a condition that primarily affects small and medium-sized arteries, which can become inflamed or damaged. This is a serious disease of the blood vessels caused by immune system malfunction. Ongoing treatment is crucial, and there is a risk of serious complications for people who have it and do not seek medical care. PAN ultimately may affect all of organs, including the skin. It can also affect the nervous system. The symptoms of PAN are likely to be quite pronounced and may include:

- Decreased appetite.
- Sudden weight loss.
- Abdominal pain.
- Excessive fatigue.
- Fever.
- Muscle and joint aches.

Yesterday, Herb was feeling down and experiencing pain in "all" of his joints. Today, he says he feels a lot better.

OK, you are the doctor. You also have your own personal problems (more complexity to confound the clinical process). Medicare hasn't increased payments and you now must adjust to lower reimbursements according to "value-based" payment schedules. With this new criteria, you will not only be required to document your activities more closely but will also be penalized if you are delinquent in reporting them. That means you will spend less time with patients. These changes bring you down, potentially infringing on your previous engaging clinical manner with patients. This level of interference is system-caused.

Identifying contributions to a clinical problem at any point in a treatment may be, as you can see, more than not easy. It may at times be close to impossible.

In this case, Herb has a central medical disorder not fully diagnosed and not yet disclosed to others. It turns out to be an autoimmune disorder later diagnosed as polyarteritis nodosa, with accompanying fevers, malaise, and painful joints. But why haven't these symptoms been reported by him? To find the answer, ask yourself whether with his anxiety and humiliation Herb is likely to acknowledge his developing medical condition and properly care for himself even if he saw a rheumatologist and received the correct diagnosis.

Undoubtedly, there is a systemic ailment here, one that is potentially progressive and may become quite serious. The complexity begins, not ends, there. Will the patient take his illness seriously? Will he follow-up and allow regular treatment. What attitude by the physician will be required to assure that the patient seeks and sustains proper care?

Little progress is likely unless his physician can "connect" with him personally as described earlier in this chapter. He does not want to acknowledge his illness and certainly seems to be compelled to minimize its impact. By staying silent, he in effect makes his disease "go away."

Personally joining with him early in treatment and engaging him in a process that is antithetical to his dismissive style would certainly have been indicated. What to do now as he pulls away, begins to close down as his physician asks for more involvement by him? Solving this kind of challenge is the strategic part of medical and psychiatric practice. An appreciation of the structure and nuances of clinical complexity is required to negotiate this process adequately.

Summary

Establishing a collaborative therapeutic relationship is often a challenge for a clinician. In this case, the patient, Herb, needed help but would not engage with his physician. His resistance was ostensibly caused by anxiety related to a chronic and progressive medical disorder that the patient was hesitant to face directly much less discuss with the clinician. The question for the clinician is how best to respond when a patient withholds critical information. Possible approaches are addressed in the next chapter.

References

1. Barber JP, Connolly MB, Crits-Christoph P, Gladis L, Siqueland L. Alliance predicts patients' outcome beyond in-treatment change in symptoms. J Consult Clin Psychol. 2000;68(6):1027–32. https://doi.org/10.1037//0022-006x.68.6.1027.
2. Brown R, Gilman A. The pronouns of power and solidarity. In: Readings in the Sociology of Language. Berlin, Boston: De Gruyter; 2012. p. 252–75.

Introduction

Some of the rudiments of establishing a treatment relationship are presented in this chapter. Facilitating this relationship may begin with the clinician judging whether a formal or informal dialogue with the patient is most likely to be productive. Next are attempts by the clinician to find areas of common ground with the patient to support their exchange of information. The "flow" of this dialogue does not necessarily follow a script and is at least partially dependent on therapeutic rapport. In the best of circumstances, the treater discerns what it is like to be that patient and strives to "get into" the patient's mind. In our experience, this effort requires authenticity on the part of both patient and clinician. In our view, steps in engaging a patient ideally include a profound and self-revealing sequence led by the clinician. The objective is for the patient to get to know the clinician as a human being who may become important in shaping his or her life.

Establishing a Treatment Relationship

Seth and Mr. G. are an unlikely pair. How do you group them? What attracted them to my practice? They were aware that I am essentially a "general practice" psychiatrist with specialty training in both general and child psychiatry, and a lot of experience treating families. Nonetheless, there is little to explain how these people decided to seek treatment from me except perhaps my reputation as a well-trained and flexible clinician.

While I am not personally so easy going, I am flexible perhaps to an unusual degree in my practice. Start with the way I introduce myself. In response to the usual, "Hello doctor," I generally respond with "feel free to call me Steve." I explain that I'd rather be called by my first name since it is likely to decrease the personal distance between us.

I have started with new patients for 40 years, insisting always on taking a history but doing it in a (deliberately) scattered-seeming way, following lines of inquiry that seem most pertinent to the patient's needs. For example, when I asked a new patient where she grew up and she said Brooklyn, I smiled and said, "I think I've heard of that place." I paused and then added that that I grew up in the Bronx (as you can probably tell by the remaining vestiges of my New York accent). So, we started by having something in common.

Soon we are comfortable enough for me to begin with the "hard questions." This is usually a tricky transition. So, when I sense that I'm beginning to step on the patient's toes, I may back off with "sounds important, but we should get to that later."

I continue with, "Let me explain how this process actually works. Everyone has their private areas and for us to deal with these effectively, you will need to share much of that information with me. Psychiatric work of this sort is … needs to be … a two-way street."

Am I applying a formula in following this sequence? Are my responses "scripted?" I do not think so. I am continually using my intuition, and plenty of it. There are verbal and nonverbal clues about the patient's level of "connection" with me, how much she hears and the associated question of how much she takes in and wants to share.

Fundamentally, I am the doctor and my clinical goal is to join with this patient so that she will want to work with me to understand and join with me in a mutually formulated treatment plan. Even better, I want the patient to collaborate with me to create or modify that plan and confirm its value. After all, it is hardly worth your time as a clinician if your patient cannot join with you.

Now that you've had the "blow-by-blow," it is time to summarize the principles. If you like what I have done, you may want to try something similar. The following is the sequence I follow. It should be generalizable to other one-to-one clinical situations:

1. I "size up" this patient looking for clues about her needs, sensibilities, and mood. I search for demographic and background information first. But that action might have trivialized the precious, groundbreaking first minutes of our contact.
2. I intuit what this patient wants to know about who I am. Should I remain formal and keep my emotional distance? This is preferable with some patients but the "kiss of death" with others.
3. I explain my tentativeness about asking personal questions early in our work. This is in effect a unilateral statement about my style implying that I will not "barge" into the patient's private life and that she will have some control over how aggressive I will be in getting information.

Even a sequence this short can have a remarkable array of interpersonal possibilities. These, of course, reflect the unique personalities of the patient and clinician and the two in combination, just as they bear a tight relationship to the patient's disease and its experienced urgency. The style I am describing is intended to convey that I believe the patient and I are on equal footing as human beings, that I want us to relate on that basis.

As a primary care physician or specialist, you may not feel you have the time to be so methodical or collaborative. But you can hardly avoid it. Think of what might happen if the patient simply is seeking a quick fix that emphasizes medication when she enters your door, and you begin by assuming she wants a definitive assessment and personal treatment. She will be out of that door before even getting started. You first need to ascertain the patient's immediate needs and tolerances, and build, if you can, toward a more precise understanding of the patient's actual wants and needs.

With this model of therapeutic action, you have a dramatic reversal of the blank screen model that at one time dominated psychiatric treatment. If this reference seems archaic to you, sample how many clinicians, medical and nonmedical, refrain from revealing themselves under the guise of "professionalism." Granted, most clinicians are cordial, interested in personally connecting with their patients. They are typically willing to share a bit about their personal lives, e.g., where they were born and their children's ages. Some consider this nonprofessional, but probably not most. Most also know intuitively that they get better cooperation from patients who find them personally accessible.

Being collaborative is an attractive ideal. It does not, however, necessarily refer to a style that is continually warm and engaging. The level and type of engagement in any treatment, medical or psychological, needs to evolve collaboratively, and the ground rules for interaction will develop accordingly. The treatment process involves what in effect is a complicated negotiation between two separate people, and the main criterion that should apply to evaluate the success is outcome. At the same time, a successful treatment process needs to be vital and creative.

There are vast areas of interpersonal connection not covered in this conventional model of professional behavior. How likely are you as a clinician to confide in someone you do not really know? Would you tell them about your sex life, whether you had ever been cited for driving under the influence of drugs or alcohol, or whether you cheat on your taxes? Yet this kind of transparency applied to personal and medical matters is often critical for getting an accurate response from another person, e.g., a patient. Certainly, these are topics that often have a critical place in a medical history. It took me years to tell my primary care physician that my mother committed suicide. I worried that my reputation as a physician could be damaged if my colleagues knew this about this fact.

What kind of violence is done to a treatment relationship (medical or not) if transparency is limited? Can you really treat a falsified patient, especially if you as the clinician are not transparent? Achieving the described level of authenticity may be beyond the reach and even desire of many, if not most, clinicians. The key question is, but what do you lose if it is absent?

What model for treatment is being recommended here? We call the described activity "the leap of inference." The discomfort achieved is intended to be *generative*, to bring either or both parties beyond the confines of their accustomed reality. "Leaps of inference" as they accumulate in the treatment process are anything but random. They may start with arbitrary choices of statements or actions. However, the result is an intervention created by either or both the clinician and patient.

In the earlier example, involving Juliana's move from her vacation home, "the leap of inference" was recognizing that Seth and Juliana both needed someone to override Seth's wife's treachery and to stop her from conspiring to break apart the family into which she had married. With Nafi (Chapter 19), it was my willingness to radically revise my long-held view of him and his character that apparently made the difference. Both instances required a dramatic revision of my initial impression of the patient and my orchestrating a therapeutic collaboration to implement my revised impressions. The direction of the treatments included my acknowledging Seth's wife's intrigue in the first example and reevaluating my obtuseness about Nafi in the second example. Most striking and inexplicable were the magnitude of the changes that resulted and the fact that changes occurred without my understanding the exact mechanisms in either case.

Summary

This chapter focuses on SAF's approach for discovering information that facilitates (a) therapeutic discovery, (b) formulation of the problems needing to be addressed, and (c) the selection of the best approach for treating a patient. Such goals require intuition about formality of approach as well as the timing of inquiry. In judging this point, recall that all medical patients need to have a formal evaluation that includes a mental status evaluation and review of systems.

Further Reading: Collaborative Treatment

Developing a collaborative working relationship. In: Systematic treatment of persistent psychosis (STOPP). CRC Press; 2002. p. 19–32.

Ciechanowski PS, Russo JE, Katon WJ, Von Korff M, Simon GE, Lin EHB, et al. The association of patient relationship style and outcomes in collaborative care treatment for depression in patients with diabetes. Med Care. 2006;44(3):283–91.

Jagosh J, Donald Boudreau J, Steinert Y, Macdonald ME, Ingram L. The importance of physician listening from the patients' perspective: enhancing diagnosis, healing, and the doctor-patient relationship. Patient Educ Couns. 2011;85(3):369–74.

Walter S, Hrabal V, Kahle J, Geibel M-A, Frisch S, Jerg-Bretzke L. Partnership and emotional support in the doctor-patient relationship–a comparison of patient preferences from 1996/1997 versus 2018. Dtsch Arztebl Int. 2021;118(23):405–6.

Engaging the Clinical Field: Introduction to Our Interpersonal Model for Change

18

Introduction

Adding to the vagaries of the clinical situation is the quality of the bond between clinician and patient. Our model holds that for treatment to be most effective, the clinician needs to reach deeply "into" the patient's thinking and emotions (in effect that person's sense of his or her "reality"). This process requires mutual transparency between treater and patient. In this exchange, the initiator is positioned to discover personal qualities in the other and in the treatment relationship that were hitherto not apparent. Our model of therapeutic change requires that the clinician (and often the patient) lose themselves in this process, a process that mandates transparency on both sides.

The next step requires patient and clinician to engage in what can be a wrenching process of self-reflection and/or self-revelation (sharing one's private thoughts and experiences with the other). Leading with almost complete transparency, the clinician acknowledges that he or she does not (fully) understand the patient and lets him/herself be "drawn into" that person's experience ("reality"). The objective is immersion by the clinician in the patient's experience and, equally, transparency on the part of the clinician in reporting his or her (often profound) response to the patient. As a clinician, you do not have genuine "access" to the patient until this process is fully engaged.

This experience often builds to the point of profound discomfort for clinician and, at times, both clinician and patient. Ultimately, exiting from this state is likely to feel confusing or even "unreal" since substantial change in the clinician or both clinician and patient has likely occurred.

One needs to actively negotiate this process, not wait for change to occur. At times, personal change may begin to take hold almost immediately. Or, its onset

---

Clinical Illustrations: Matthew (17-year-old boxer), Otto (19-year-old and developmentally disabled), and Lex (55-year-old entrepreneur).

© The Author(s), under exclusive license to Springer Nature Switzerland AG 2023
S. A. Frankel et al., *Complexity in Health Care*,
https://doi.org/10.1007/978-3-031-14949-8_18

may be delayed creating the impression that progress is not occurring. We call the technique of exploiting disunity between clinician and patient for the purpose of making clinical progress a "leap of inference" [1]. To be effective, the "leap of inference" requires that clinician and/or patient depart from previous convictions about each other and their expectations for how the treatment process will unfold. Note that this assault on one's familiar sense of how treatment should be conducted and its probable outcome is often neither expected nor understood. That personal change has occurred is often surprising to either or both participants.

My Approach to the Patient (SAF)

I join with the patient, no superiority, dogged transparency, but contained so I do not invite distortions about my motivations. I am insistently self-reflective, often sharing my personal reflections with the patient, always concerned about the clinical consequences of what (the ideas and emotions) I introduce. I share what I have come to believe are my insights about the patient's motivations and deeper needs, but only after testing the validity of these with the patient. I have become vigorous with instigating "leaps of inference." I jump in when after repeated attempts I believe that for defensive reasons (or because I'm wrong) the patient, like Nafi whose story is developed below, does not understand my intent.

Additionally, I often find myself deeply empathizing with aspects of the patient (his or her life, ambitions, values, accomplishments, struggles) that I respect or admire.

Here, I am likely to "flip" to the patient's side since with my shift in comprehension, I have come to see the "truth" in the patient's convictions. I find areas of "brilliance" in patients who were previously distinguished by their limitations and *modify my theory of the patient's psychology* to fit. Examples include Otto, who at age 20 was referred to me as "developmentally disabled and intermittently psychotic," and Lex, 55-years-old, whose intellectual brilliance and personal vulnerability made it hard for people to understand and sometimes tolerate him. I often find myself powerfully attaching to these people and advocating for them. This maneuver has the distinct benefit of identifying and emphasizing that patient's unique attributes and in many instances demarcating the point around which personal change will be initiated. Also, this action is often powerful for engaging the patient to cooperate with the treatment.

Here is an unlikely scenario illustrating this process with 17-year-old Matthew, an aspiring boxer. What *really* mattered to him was imagining himself risking his life as a member of one of the US Army Special Forces. I have never been attracted by idealized versions of masculinity. In fact, one of my proudest achievements was being granted conscientious objector status in my late adolescence. The result was that if called to serve I would have entered the military as a "medic." Yet Matthew intrigued me. The book he recommended on "snipers" was hideous, but 17-year-old Matthew seemed heroic as I watched the bloody videos he sent me of himself sparring with older boxers. I, of course, could understand why he might have chosen boxing as his sport. He had been unendingly harassed by his older brother. But my genuine fondness for him was inexplicable and the product of our personal "connection." I was inspired by his convictions. How strange for a 78-year-old man to be inspired by a 17-year-old boy. It makes me think of the yearbook inscriptions from high school, "don't ever change." Honestly, I felt like saying that to Matthew despite, but maybe because of, our profound differences.

Otto

The process described was similar for Otto and Lex. Otto, age 19, was a "goner." Everyone but his parents had given up on him. He was regarded as intellectually and socially "retarded" by teachers and students, and he was always academically and socially behind his agemates, usually by large increments.

Otto's big personal struggle at that moment was to get enough marijuana to "party" each day. But he had been presented to me as sweetly naive. Remarkably enough his "sweetness" morphed into cleverness in concocting advanced ways to fenagle his parents into supplying anything he wanted, including marijuana. Fast forward and our pathetic, "impaired" subject changes into a "smooth operator." Working with him in treatment, rather than being a torment, turned out to be fascinating. Otto methodically taught me how remarkably adaptable, how clever, an "intellectually impaired" person could be.

Lex

It was the opposite with Lex, 55-years-old, and renown in his field as a financial "whiz," a "ground breaking thinker." He had been to the finest universities and prided himself on the quickness and accuracy of his thinking. The problem was that his relationships would fall apart and his closest associates, most particularly his wife, regularly took advantage of him. Over time his wife reviled him mercilessly, and when the marriage fell apart she continued to harass him, with Lex least prepared for this. As a tribute to Lex's brilliance when he caught on to these developments, generally toward the end of an onslaught, he was able to cleverly correct the situation, vanquishing his adversary including his treacherous wife.

The fix? Lex was unusual, remarkably smart and talented. He had been in psychotherapy for years but without benefit. Logically what he needed was his own brand of treatment, one predicated on his brilliance and modified for his temperament. In both of these cases a radical reorientation of the treater and the treatment was required. The original "rules" didn't apply. New rules needed to be created.

Summary

For many clinicians, the foundation of therapeutic change is "rapport." In this chapter, rapport in the treatment relationship is extended to include not only improved understanding but also profound involvement between the two participants.

Reference

1. Frankel SA. Making psychotherapy work: collaborating effectively with your patient. London: Psychosocial Press; 2007.

Inexplicable Reversals that Facilitate Change

19

Introduction

Major shifts in treatment may be difficult to explain and predict. Two cases are used to illustrate such shifts. Case 1: An impending crisis involving a patient, his wife, and his mother, and its remarkable resolution is used for illustration. Case 2: An unexpected reversal in behavior and thinking for a second patient who had habitually refused to consider well-intentioned observations from others is described. In both cases, change was not anticipated and was inexplicable, but welcomed.

The timing of the kinds of personal change described in this chapter often is unpredictable. The ingredients are generally manifold but often their magnitude and juxtaposition with other events are obscure. In the next two examples, major developments were unanticipated and not predicted. The first example involves a remarkable instance of how change may occur on a group basis when the clinician is able to be "in the shoes" of the other participants.

Clinical Illustration: Seth and Juliana

Seth, Juliana's son, age 49, was already in deep trouble with his mother in advance of this incident. Because of his inadvertent provocations and her paranoid tendencies, he had been ousted from his originally elevated position with his mother. He typically missed emotional cues and took positions that inflamed his mother. Making matters especially tense was that Juliana had cancer that rendered her weakened and emotionally unstable.

Clinical Illustrations: (1) Seth and Juliana and (2) Nafi

© The Author(s), under exclusive license to Springer Nature Switzerland AG 2023   113
S. A. Frankel et al., *Complexity in Health Care*,
https://doi.org/10.1007/978-3-031-14949-8_19

In this incident, family members had gathered to help Juliana permanently leave the family vacation home. At first spirits were high, everyone wanting to help. However, without notice, Seth suddenly slipped away. He had gone to inspect a nearby house he and his wife had discussed buying as their second home. Everyone was shocked when his absence was revealed. To make matters worse, on return, he announced he and his wife had decided to buy this house. His decision was provocative since, because of personal conflicts, Juliana was vehemently opposed to his buying a home in that neighborhood. No one except Seth was aware of the pressure he (Seth) was experiencing from his wife to buy the new house. She was surreptitiously attempting to instigate a family mutiny based on her hostility toward Seth's mother and her wish to put a wedge between mother and son.

Once informed about Seth's intentions, Juliana became enraged. Only I (SAF), in my counseling role, was aware of how damaging the situation could be to family unity. As predicted, family members were soon at war. When queried, Seth defended himself rationalizing that his fondness for the new house was based on it being located near the now sold traditional family vacation home. He claimed (falsely) that purchasing the new house would allow him to intermittently visit the beloved family vacation home.

My job became to prevent a family debacle (Seth's wife's motive was to incite this) by joining with as many members of the family as possible. Juliana immediately started to blame Seth, alleging disloyalty, and inflaming the situation. I directed Seth's sister to temporarily take charge as mediator. I remained in my counseling role using the sister as a support while I communicated vigorously with each person except Seth's wife.

Events deteriorated with lightning speed Juliana was venomous and not willing to be appeased. Seth's wife was at the center insisting she "must have" the new house. The debacle lasted for 3 days, with everyone confused and ultimately exhausted. However, in the end, Juliana relented. She did not want to destroy family unity despite her rage. Clearly, all could have been lost, the family thrown into permanent disarray.

Nonetheless, it was remarkable to witness how rapidly Seth responded when I could clarify the psychology of the situation him. It had been 6 months since this event. Seth had been talking regularly to me and now was reconciled with Juliana. How to explain the rather remarkable turnaround of events? After recognizing the peril to the family, all members were ultimately able to reverse course, except Seth's wife. Her treachery had been contained, but barely.

This example is presented to illustrate how complicated interpersonal situations may become and how important it is for a clinician to embrace, not overlook, their complexity. Central to these events was my recognizing the danger of this situation by putting myself in Juliana's shoes as well as those of the other family members. While everything was falling apart, I found myself imagining what each member would experience if the family collapsed. The upset caused by Juliana's cancer added urgency. The threat to family survival had to be my guide, and my temporary shift in this situation was from internally taking in (internalizing) the reality of the participants.

Nafi's Inexplicable and Rapid Reversal

Nafi, age 53, was unmarried and troubled about his inability to find a wife. Nafi provides a good illustration of a dramatic clinical reversal. It is important to emphasize that the described order of interpersonal events is equally relevant in general medicine, psychiatry, and psychology.

Nafi insisted that he loved Akane, not wanting to acknowledge evidence that her behavior was erratic and more convenient than heartfelt. Nafi and I had a history of repeated confrontations based on his insistence on "doing it in his way." I had treated Nafi for a few years, both with psychotherapy and psychopharmacology, repeatedly challenging his resistance to taking suggestions from others, including myself.

In this case, I struggled to point out what I and others believed was the folly of his ill-conceived insistence about marrying Akane. But Nafi dug in. He did not want to hear my warning nor that of others. He obsessively held his ground and as predicted I soon had an emotional cripple on my hands, Akane resisting his overtures and Nafi overwhelmed with despair. Soon he could not sleep or work. Adding to Nafi's woes, his father had been diagnosed with brain cancer, glioblastoma multiforme. He had no more than a few months to live. As context, his family was the mainstay of Nafi's life.

The situation became more complicated. Nafi was simply convinced that he had to marry Akane. She soon showed her true opportunistic colors and abruptly decided to move to Hong Kong to live with another man and his two latency-age children. This man had a stunning reputation as a chef and was quite wealthy. Nafi was bereft. He could not believe that Akane could abandon their relationship and scuttle all the attention he had showered on her over their 10-year relationship. He believed that he had been entirely "selfless" in his attention to her. And now this.

Despairing, Nafi at first thought about suicide but after a few months decided to return to Pakistan to live with his 79-year-old mother who would likely survive her husband's demise. His whole life was in flames. As a physician or psychotherapist, if you allow yourself to become involved in your patients' lives, you are likely to find them asking for advice about all sorts of personal matters, many of which you are ill-equipped to handle.

At that point, Nafi also came close to firing me. He was angry about the "bad advice" I had given him. All hope seemed to be lost. In fact, as much as I could contain it, the disaffection was mutual. By that point, I was beginning to feel like I had enough of Nafi's self-righteousness. To be honest, despite my original firm commitment to our work, I was beginning to hope he would disappear.

But here is the twist. In his despondency, Nafi was slowly being forced to question his core assumptions. His self-esteem had been based on the conviction that he was simply a "nice selfless guy" and that this trait alone would gain him the rewards he firmly believed he deserved.

This all may sound ominous, endangering my work with him, but in fact, it was the kind of imbalance that can facilitate change. And, indeed, something inexplicable began to happen. It was happening to both of us.

Mind you, no manner of exhortation had been effective with Nafi. But I can remember the moment - and it was a moment - when I caught on. I cannot tell you what convinced me, but the shift within me and then in the treatment was momentous. My guess is that we both were tired of the tension between us. We were looking for something better and were silently becoming open to recognizing it. My empathy about Nafi's impending loss of his father was also at work.

In what seemed like a split second, I realized that to this point, I had been unable to shift my perception of Nafi and his motives. I apologize for sounding unscientific. Whatever intuition is, that is what was suddenly at work. It happened like a flash... and I got it! I was beginning to see that, at heart, Nafi might really be as well-meaning and generous as he claimed. I suddenly could see that he really did care about people and wanted the best for them. He simply did not know how to describe this, and to his detriment, this sentiment was often expressed through a rational argument making him seem insufferably self-righteous.

I told Nafi about my shift. He cautiously accepted it. Still, Akane intermittently returned to haunt Nafi, assuming first place in his mind. Nonetheless, something powerful was happening. Nafi was easing up, and *so was I*. We were *both* changing.

Several months later, Nafi, who had been socially isolated for years, impulsively decided to invite his work group to his home for an "ethnic dinner." This move was groundbreaking for him. When this event succeeded beyond expectation, he began to find other opportunities to get together with these people. At first, he defensively labeled these dinners as "forced."

This is a good point to reveal other information about Nafi. He had been referred to me by a friend of his who had attended graduate school in the United States with him. The friend described Nafi as unparalleled in his brilliance about financial matters. There was a lot of evidence supporting this claim. Backing it up, however, was the fact that our unprepossessing subject had made a fortune by the time he was 40. The single trauma to that point in his life had been a relationship during college that came to an unfortunate end when his girlfriend at age 20 suddenly decided to marry another man. This event haunted him up through the ill-fated relationship with Akane 25 years later.

My conviction is that recovery of this magnitude is possible, probably common but often not comprehended. Building up to it may be paradox, contradiction, and disappointments that may each look end-stage. Patients and clinicians may be inclined to give up at any point, and not necessarily at the same times. Money and personal support may run out, ending the ordeal as failure.

But I insist. This kind of "magical" healing occurs more frequently than is commonly appreciated. It, of course, must have ingredients contributed both by clinician and patient. But, given all the writing that has been done on personal change through medical and psychotherapeutic treatment, could the magic soup here really be as simple as understanding, empathy, and shared respect, as well as the interpersonal sequence detailed in the last chapter? Maybe not always, but in some cases, likely. After all, there is a lot written (see Barber and Muran, Chapter 12) about the treatment alliance and its central role in treatment adherence as well as symptom cure and personal change.

Summary

The case studies of Seth (and his mother, Juliana) and Nafi have been presented to illustrate unexpected events that (a) contribute to patient complexity and (b) can become integral in producing change.

Further Reading: Unexpected and Unexplained Change Associated with Clinical Work

Fainzang S, Hem HE, Risor MB. The taste for knowledge: Medical anthropology facing medical realities. Aarhu: Aarhus University Press; 2010.

Nissen N, Bech Risør M. Diagnostic fluidity: Working with uncertainty and mutability. Publicacions Universitat Rovira i Virgili; 2018.

Part IX

Treatment, Including Review of Cases

[Part Introduction: In this part of the book, we collect and examine our case examples for the purpose of expanding our understanding of clinical complexity. What commonalities can we identify among these cases apart from the fact that they are complicated in structure and typically involve complex patients? Do they require extra time and/or resources to manage? Are the treatment teams required to manage them inherently different than those required for more typical cases?]

20

Complexity in Treatment of Complex Versus Routine Clinical Situations

Introduction

In this chapter, case studies are revisited to illustrate clinical complexity that was at first not appreciated by the clinician. Sifting through the multitude of variables in the clinical situation is a challenging task for the clinician. Procedures using abductive reasoning and algorithms to accomplish this task are discussed.

Reviewing our case examples highlights the variation in and disparate nature of the factors (variables) governing clinical work. It is not that this finding is a surprise, but it does admonish us as clinicians to maintain humility about how well and with what depth we understand clinical situations and to remind us of the potential imprecision of our clinical judgments.

Here we will present case illustrations that demonstrate systemic-medical, psychiatric, social, cultural, and interpersonal complexity. We will also highlight multiple perspectives associated with clinical work, e.g., patient, physician, population (public health), and how each influences the evolving case formulation and treatment. Subtle, frequently unacknowledged, factors will be highlighted.

Medical information from and decisions by physicians often represent approximations in part because of the time, expense, and sophistication required to collect and process the information available. For these reasons, clinicians are often compelled to leave out and conflate details. They may do this by using heuristic methods, including diagnostic categories and algorithms to summarize the patient's clinical condition, rather than expounding on actual clinical details. Including the patient's, the clinician's, and at times public health perspectives represents clinical work as it is and as it evolves, creating the basis for the assessment and the treatment approaches we develop throughout this book.

© The Author(s), under exclusive license to Springer Nature Switzerland AG 2023 121
S. A. Frankel et al., *Complexity in Health Care*,
https://doi.org/10.1007/978-3-031-14949-8_20

Understanding Clinical Events Abductively (Probabilistically) from Case Material

What makes organizing and treating complex cases so difficult? Apart from providing needed medical and personal resources (time and expertise), how can a clinician improve his or her effort in these situations? Rigorously developed algorithms are the most common recourse for finding one's way. Nonetheless, treatments using these summary methods often fail to accurately capture the clinical situation.

Outside of our published research, our data to this point in the book comes from case illustrations and experience. Cases so far include Mr. G., Seth and his family including Juliana (two illustrations), Mark (diabetic), Luke and Boris (the two 35-year-old men who appeared superficially similar), Jasmine (the woman from Yemen with schizophrenia), Beth (the diabetic woman), Herb (polyarteritis nodosa), Nafi, and the new patient making her first office visit, 17-year-old Matthew, and 20-year-old Otto.

What are the systemic medical and other pathology-related factors that are common to these examples? What are the less appreciated contributions? Here is a short list taken from our examples:

- Anxiety deflecting from compliance with assessment and treatment (e.g., Mark, Herb).
- Interpersonal conflict as it affects patient compliance and/or family cooperation (e.g., Seth, Juliana).
- Imprecise or incorrect diagnostic labels (e.g., Jasmine; Luke and Boris).
- Cultural impediments (e.g., Mr. G. and Jasmine).
- The patient not understanding his or her illness, with lack of understanding impeding cooperation with practitioners (e.g., Mark).
- Conflict between the practitioner's goals and the patient's (e.g., Nafi).
- "Mystery," i.e., clinical factors that still need to be clarified. As with Nafi, variables influencing compliance and outcome are often elusive and at the time of presentation not yet understood.
- Developmental factors (e.g., 17-year-old Matthew, 20-year-old Otto).

Since these contributions can skew one's clinical formulation and exclusion of any of them from a treatment design can impair patient compliance and treatment success, how can the most relevant items be identified and incorporated into treatment? Physicians may attempt to do this by using formulas (algorithms) and intuitively using experience as their guide.

Mr. G.'s case illustrates interference with treatment from patient noncompliance. Mr. G. felt that his security was not guaranteed when he was in the hands of an American doctor. His solution was to withhold facts about his medical history, analogous to his need to protect his identity from his Taliban captors during wartime. He was beset with post-traumatic stress disorder (PTSD) and chronically anxious about real and imagined risks associated with cooperation with American doctors. When he was hired at a major convenience store to drive a forklift, he was so distracted by anxiety that he hit and injured a customer. Reflective of his distrust, he withheld payments from his doctor, lying about family support for his medical care and financial competency. In the end, he was "fired" by both his physician and employer. While a behavioral designation, lack of compliance, is illustrated here, PTSD and paranoia more accurately and less pejoratively capture the fundamental clinical issues. Consequently, there were a range of treatments for his practitioner to consider including (1) a therapeutically relevant exploration of Mr. G.'s background, (2) a careful emotionally guided review of the events of his trauma, (3) cognitive behavioral therapy including desensitization, and (4) medication.

Next consider Herb (also see Chapter 16), the man who hid his physical deterioration from his employer and wife. The manifestations included at first undisclosed and unexplained joint pains, fever, and weight loss. These clinical manifestations as a group are consistent with malignancies and a myriad of autoimmune diseases. The precursors of these conditions may be unrecognized, initially masquerading as another condition, e.g., fibromyalgia. We now know the cause of the symptoms he tried to hide. Polyarteritis nodosa is a rare, serious, progressive condition. Hiding one's condition does no good; the disease will stay and move along even though it may be a long time before a definitive diagnosis can be made. You can see how difficult complexity factors, especially those that are subjective, may be to organize and prioritize in case formulations and treatment plans. For example, how to rate the importance of Herb's anxiety, denial, and embarrassment and where to place these in an assessment and treatment scheme?

Further Reading: Abductive Thinking (Creativity in Clinical Work)

Gabbay DM, Smets P. Abductive Reasoning and Learning. Dordrecht, Netherlands: Springer; 2000.
Liberatore P, Schaerf M. On the complexity of second-best abductive explanations. Int J Approximate Reason. 2015;63:22–31.
Walton D. Abductive reasoning. Tuscaloosa, AL: University of Alabama Press; 2014.

Treatment: Clinical Details

21

Introduction

This chapter explicates issues of diagnosis and treatment for a complex cancer patient, Maggie. Involved in her care was a team of medical specialists. Her active social and professional life had been disrupted by cancer and painful medical interventions. Of importance is the indignity she experienced as the sequela to multiple medical/surgical interventions (e.g., chronic, excruciating pain; a "disgusting" colostomy). The chapter ends with the topic of treatment team management.

In this chapter, we illustrate how inconsequential-seeming factors, in Maggie's case an assault on her dignity, can be a primary consideration for understanding a patient's treatment needs and formulating an intervention. For example, a patient may be disrupted by forced life changes. This kind of disruption is often unexpected and can be personally catastrophic for the patient and family. Its impact may equal or even override the associated medical considerations.

For Herb, creation of a treatment plan was disrupted by factors associated with his anxiety about having a disease, and perhaps more centrally by his masculine pride.

Maggie: A Complicated Case

Maggie had vaginal cancer. Side effects from chemotherapy had been "intolerable" and included excruciating pelvic and labial (external) pain. This ordeal had been going on for months, and while the chemotherapeutic agent she was treated with resulted in the remission of her cancer, she was in constant pain. She could hardly sit comfortably for more than a few minutes. In the previous month, she also required a colostomy which she said was "awful to manage, unpleasant, and disgusting."

Clinical illustration: Maggie, an Elderly Woman with Vaginal Cancer

S. A. Frankel et al., *Complexity in Health Care*, https://doi.org/10.1007/978-3-031-14949-8_21

Medical management, including pain control, was challenging enough in this case. But "dignity management" (our term) for this once proud woman was equally pertinent. Previously, Maggie entertained the socially elite of her community and lived a "very public life." The world "was always at my fingertips." For other people, clinical complexity may oppositely pivot around financial disadvantage. An interesting feature of this case is that affluence was problematic since decorum was so essential in Maggie's circles. Her condition made it difficult for her to maintain her dignity. For example, her colostomy made gurgling noises that anyone could hear, and she felt mortified as a result.

Ordinarily, a physician might approach a case like this as follows. Using available information, the initial assessment and early intervention may take up to 6 months and include history, examinations, referrals to specialists focused on oncology, laboratory work, diagnostic scans, and surgery. Accompanying this process is the challenging task of delivering to the patient with (as she put it) "the most terrible news I have ever received," plans for the next period of her life going up in smoke.

Maggie's husband was about to retire, and they planned to take the "cruise of a lifetime." Suddenly, her life was split into (at least) two major segments, *personal* (including plans and ambitions) and *medical* (consisting of unending medical appointments including those intended for her maintenance and rehabilitation). Her meticulously planned life would be "thoroughly disrupted." As a successful lawyer, her life had been highly (and "satisfactorily") structured with the help of two full-time assistants.

A patient, in her predicament, will commonly be joined by friends, parents, and children, as well as medical and self-proclaimed "experts." Most likely, each one will have a point of view about how to understand and manage her newly discovered cancer. There are likely to be recommendations about diet, exercise, nonmedical supplements, and spiritual guidance. In Maggie's case, the oncologist had no enthusiasm for any of these modalities. While spiritual support might help personally, the oncologist held that it would have no medical impact. The oncologist had a fine reputation, was familiar with all recent medical advances, but was not interested in discussing these "unsubstantiated" measures. Maggie's daughter, who herself was a cancer survivor, attributed her own recovery to the influence of a spiritual figure who had supported her throughout her illness. She unrelentingly pressed her point of view with Maggie, compounding Maggie's consternation.

Team Management

Switch now to team management where specialists collaborate under direction of one or more leader who creates a treatment plan with input from team members. The plan is supported through reference to medical literature and "best" medical practice. In this case, the team met weekly with 15 minutes allocated for discussing each patient. There was a consultant and intermittent contact with the chief of medicine through the team leader, with administrators monitoring utilization.

Interdisciplinary Team Management

22

Introduction

This chapter continues with the complex case of Maggie. Emphasis is on the functioning of a multidisciplinary treatment team. Recall that Maggie was an aging patient who, following medical interventions for cancer, continued to experience extreme pain. Involved were repeated pelvic surgeries that included a colostomy. Maggie was also dissatisfied with her clinicians. Effective team management requires organization, cooperation, and efficient leadership. In Maggie's case, a lack of cohesion in the treatment team added significantly to the overall case complexity. The chapter ends with delineation of a model of treatment management.

Treatment in difficult clinical cases generally requires team management, with practitioners from various disciplines involved. Complexities may involve lack of coordination among team members and lapses in team leadership. In Maggie's case, her suffering and discontent and the lack of cooperation among team members seriously complicated the treatment process.

Intervention: Continued

In this chapter, we again make the case that inconsequential seeming factors can significantly influence clinical work and should not be overlooked. In the following sections, we discuss the issue of developing a treatment plan by organizing and prioritizing both obvious and subtle treatment variables. In Herb's case, this process with the tentative diagnosis of polyarteritis nodosa initially included a history, electromyography to rule out peripheral neuropathy, and laboratory tests for inflammation such as C-reactive protein. Angiography came later. His attitude throughout, however, was to minimize his symptoms.

Clinical illustration: Maggie (2)

© The Author(s), under exclusive license to Springer Nature Switzerland AG 2023   127
S. A. Frankel et al., *Complexity in Health Care*,
https://doi.org/10.1007/978-3-031-14949-8_22

Team Management

Team management, especially for complex patients/cases is a collaborative process. The inclusion of several professionals and/or care delivery systems is typical. In this chapter, we examine this additional layer of complexity (multiple individual professionals, treatment team), and the often subtle social and interpersonal factors that are influential in these situations.

A practitioner needs to be discerning. But it is not enough for the clinician to follow rules of "best practice." From the patient's point of view, the treatment must work and symptoms need to resolve. It is common for a clinician to be misguided about diagnosis and/or treatment and the person most likely to first catch on is the patient. How many times have you heard: "the doctor got it wrong," alluding to misdiagnosis of which the patient is likely to be uniquely aware of when symptoms persist?

It would be nice if team treatment were so straightforward consisting of competent team leadership, cooperative members, and a smooth treatment process. But the history of Maggie's team provides a realistic contrast. Team members came from different disciplines, including social work, nursing, and psychiatry. The case manager was an advanced practice registered nurse (APRN). Maggie's psychiatrist, well trained in psychotherapy, was on the periphery, but the case manager had little experience with psychiatry and almost none with psychotherapy. Early on, the oncologist became impatient with the patient's nurse advocate, repeatedly claiming that her presence was inappropriate and bothersome. The team leader, the nurse case manager, was efficient but not well organized, often losing track of individual team members.

Maggie, Continued

Changing Locations: Making matters more difficult, the location of the clinical operation had to be shifted from the local medical center to a distant major medical center because of medical insurance restrictions. The case manager and oncologist remained but other team members did not. Meanwhile, Maggie's personal situation was becoming increasingly intolerable. She began to talk about "giving up," her quality of life having "so thoroughly deteriorated."

Maggie's Condition gets Worse: Maggie's situation was medically and personally dire, at least according to Maggie. Maggie was despondent, flaring up at anyone who claimed they could help her with irascible comments like "I want to die, just leave me alone." Meanwhile, her medical situation continued to deteriorate, but not because of malignant lesions. She developed a fistula between her bowel and vagina as an unwanted effect of radiation treatments, leading to constant leakage of fluid through her vagina. She needed nursing attention and, more particularly, psychiatric care. Her children were on edge, as was her private nurse. The conversation with her psychiatrist became more like that between a hospice nurse and patient, reflecting Maggie's disconsolation. According to Maggie, since there was "no hope" (in her mind), she had "no choice" other than to prepare to die. She withdrew, relying strictly on opioids for relief of the painful inflammation in her pelvic area.

Follow-Up

Things were rough for her psychiatrist also. He dreaded his twice weekly visits with Maggie. At this point, there was mutual repulsion between them, and the team had started to see the management of the case as hopeless.

The irony of this situation is that Maggie's most recent pelvic scan showed no evidence of cancer recurrence. It was just that her symptoms derived from her radiation treatments were so constant and painful and were taken by her as a signal to give up, raising the question for the team treatment of how they should function in this situation. That Maggie might go on living cancer-free was no longer being entertained by Maggie, the oncologist being the chief naysayer defending the idea that cancer seemed to be contained.

It is worth letting you in on the fact that 3 years later, Maggie was still cancer-free. Her moods were still volatile. She vacillated between believing she could survive and wanting to throw in the towel. Adding to the confusion, she decided that one local oncological consultant was "worthless" and the other was "OK."

An Appropriate Treatment Model

So what treatment model is most applicable for this (interpersonally) complex but not unusual case?

- What about "collaborative care?" *The Collaborative Care Model* involves a psychiatrist who, in coordination with a case manager, acts as consultant to a treatment team that includes a psychiatric care/case manager [1]. This model of care would free the system from having to provide a psychiatrist on a regular basis. How could a consulting physician understand this patient in any other than a superficial way with so little personal and historical information available? In that case, the patient will quickly be passed back to the care of her PCP.
- *Stepped Care*, involving transfers to different levels of care, is another alternative. But in that case, continuity may be missing, the patient transferred from one level of care (generally from one clinic to another) to the next.

In truth, all models currently available may involve a defect in continuity within or between systems. All the models are in some way incomplete, since they can only supply a fraction of what the patient seeks in addition to competent medical care, e.g., committed treatment where the physician knows the patient well and can demonstrate that he or she personally cares about the patient's welfare. While this way of thinking may seem impractical, research on the treatment process highlights the importance of care continuity to satisfactory outcome.

This point of view recalls my (SAF) experience in South Africa years ago at the height of apartheid. That medical system had virtually no skilled personnel and very limited medical supplies. Residents of these severely under-resourced areas, called "townships," had very few bathrooms at their disposal, jobs were extraordinarily scarce, and health measures were primitive. They needed to devise something better: AIDS was rampant, afflicting over half the population. Their remarkable solution was to recruit grandmothers (men were in short supply and most were HIV positive; many were close to death) and organize them into community resource groups. These enterprising women divided up neighborhoods and organized themselves to care for children and young adults. And it worked! These denizens of the earth knew the importance of committed, caring relationships. Their university was their neighborhood, and their research participants were their own children.

Reference

1. Unutzner J, Harbin H, Schoenbaum M. The collaborative Care Model: an approach for integrating physical and mental health care. Baltimore, MD: HEALTH HOME Information Resource Center; 2013.

Further Reading: Interdisciplinary, Collaborative Teams

Chiocchio F, Kelloway EK, editors. Psychology and management of project teams: an interdisciplinary perspective. Cary, NC: Oxford University Press; 2015.
Nancarrow S, Booth A, Roots A. Ten principles of good interdisciplinary team work. Hum Resour Health. 2013;11:19.

Part X

Assessment in Clinically Complex Situations

[Part Introduction: Medical, assessments, including psychiatric, psychological, and neuropsychological require precision. Tools available to conduct these assessments include those based on mathematics and statistics. Mathematics utilizes measurement and statistical probability, e.g., the likelihood that an event will occur, that a proposition is true, or that two or more events are correlated. Methods for statistically and mathematically formalizing complex clinical situations have been developed, but they tend to be cumbersome, e.g., utilizing scores from an empirical study to organize and evaluate demographic data. In this part, we review methods for finding, collecting, and making sense out of complicated clinical data.]

Introduction

Assessment based on our revised clinical paradigm begins with a detailed (narrative) description of the patient. These data may be organized to conform to a process analogous to the statistical technique called "factor analysis," where correlated variables are grouped together as "factors." In this version of our procedure variables that display interrelationships (correlations) can be treated as similar in nature, thus simplifying the unstable intricacies of the patient's clinical situation. Case illustrations using this technique are presented in this and following chapters.

Cases summarized formally through nomothetic conventions such as diagnostic categories are in effect falsified. These versions may be anemic renderings of the actual clinical situation. The two patients described in this chapter suffered as a result of this kind of simplification, not receiving the full treatment they required.

At this point in the book, we are progressively arriving at a revised clinical model for understanding and managing complex clinical situations. It is based on patient and clinician regularly reconfiguring their understanding of and approach to the current clinical situation. What subtle clinical factors comprise this model and how do these improve outcome? The clinical narratives below help us explore these issues.

In the next two chapters, we look at the two basic approaches for formulating clinical data, narrative (idiographic), and research (group data, nomothetic) and how they can enhance one another. As an example, consider a patient whose experience of abuse in childhood is conceptually linked to depressive disorder and fear of doctors as an adult (idiographic) vs. the same person who using validated screening tools based on group data is identified as not compliant with medications in adulthood (nomothetic). Citing "data" that is both narrative and research-based leads

---

Clinical illustrations: Two highly accomplished people each with significant depression— (1) A despondent woman who commits suicide and (2) Ben, depression leading to paralysis

© The Author(s), under exclusive license to Springer Nature Switzerland AG 2023
S. A. Frankel et al., *Complexity in Health Care*,
https://doi.org/10.1007/978-3-031-14949-8_23

to a fuller appreciation of a clinical situation than when findings are based on either method alone. We will present (1) narratives that illustrate how clinical formulations are arrived at ideographically and (2) the contrasting-complementary contribution of research data, i.e., nomothetic. How do the two approaches add to each other and how might they lead to different conclusions/clinical approaches? What are the problems and advantages associated with using either method alone to guide work with complex patients/cases?

Case Narratives Compared to Formal, "Evidence-Based" Reports

When explicating clinical complexity, we need to identify the essence of each case including diagnoses and central pathophysiological dysfunctions, i.e., the patient's physiological, metabolic, and biochemical derangements combined with the ongoing impact of the environment on the development of the case. These are the bedrock on which the patient's clinical existence is scaffolded. There is no more inclusive way to illustrate this complicated, shifting configuration than with ongoing, detailed case narratives. Of course, you may ask why we as scientists should be comfortable with case narratives (invariably reported through the filter of subjectivity). The final narrative is a composite of all the elements named: medical facts, pertinent personal information, social and sociological contributions, and the clinician's experience, preferences, and prejudices. Chronologically, this evolving process is longitudinal, extending from the start of treatment. It incorporates the financial capabilities of the subject/project as they evolve. For this complicated matrix of factors (variables) to be managed, it must be simplified, variables correlated, and numbers of variables reduced. This process is like the statistical procedure called "factor analysis." Factor analysis (and its relative, structural equation modeling) is discussed later in this book.

Probably, the only way to represent the "real" clinical picture with maximum accuracy is through narrative. But, of course, narratives are usually manipulated so they can be focused and to make intended points. You know this. It is basic stuff. But how often have you thought about what is eliminated or simplified when a case is discussed? The rendering generally includes either too much or too little, leaving a middle ground that must be carefully reconstructed so the case is minimally fabricated.

Case 1, Suicide
Here is an example of a clinical narrative for a complex patient. Imagine that your mother (who for the purpose of this presentation we will call "Mother") is admitted to the hospital for an unspecified condition. The physician, who seems astute and humane, comes to you (her daughter) and says her liver function tests are moderately abnormal and her cognition (recall and orientation) seems slightly compromised. Somewhere in the back of your mind you recall being told that when your mother was younger, she worked in a factory and was exposed to toxic chemicals. As an adolescent, she also reportedly had a "mild" case of poliomyelitis, which was

epidemic in the 1940s. Indeed, she developed as slight limp as a sequelae. Add that she is 82-years-old and prone to depression.

We now have some of the main medical facts of her case. Not included is that consistent with her early history of illness, she is constantly petrified about dying. Each new pain elicits a new story of a disease she believes she has. Her son says that when he was 5 years old, her anxiety became so intense that she was hospitalized three times, twice for episodes diagnosed as pancreatitis (although her blood lipase and amylase were within normal limits throughout the hospitalizations).

Maybe this is not such a big deal. It is not so unusual for people to present with abdominal pain of "unknown origin." In those cases, there is often a suspicion that the pain is emotionally based (indicative of a "somatic symptom disorder"), but the possibility that the pain is the harbinger of a yet unidentified medical condition makes it imperative to take it seriously.

We now have some of the main medical facts of her case. Not included is that each new pain elicits a new story of a disease she believes she probably has.

Unfortunately, she did not do well. Wracked by pain, the patient was unnerved by the absence of definitive findings. Her physician prescribed barbiturates. Dependent on these for relief, the patient began to withdraw from her previous active life. Old friends withdrew as well, disbelieving her claim of pancreatitis. Once beautiful, she progressively lost weight, her appearance rapidly deteriorating. Her son had left for college, deeply troubled by what was happening to his mother but unable to help. She took a job working in partnership with an old friend but had a vicious argument that soon ended the friendship. Meanwhile, Julia, her physician, kept prescribing barbiturates. Her son returned from college for the summer to find his mother slurring her words. She was admitted to the hospital again: something about "adhesions" and the pain being "unbearable." She would sit in the bathroom for hours expelling massive amounts of "gas." The point here is that things worsened rapidly giving the impression of a progressing medical condition. This once beautiful, intellectually gifted woman became physically crippled and unattractive both physically and personally.

It was not just her son who found the patient repulsive. It was her husband as well. Soon, there was no one to monitor or correct this situation. The second son was also in college and had secretly eloped with a hometown girl, eliciting his father's ire and his mother's grief. The patient's husband began to have a romantic affair with a colleague.

Wait. Stop for a moment. Did not this all start with abdominal pain? The family had been "tight," "stable." The father was a teacher at a prestigious public school. The older son was vice president of his high school class and in competition for being the valedictorian. The younger son was equally, if not more, promising, besting his brother by being both an athlete and scholar. Originally, the picture was that of a mother presiding over a "perfect" family. There was an illness of undetermined origin that included repetitive episodes of pain. And then mother's questionable physical and clear-cut psychological collapse, including eventual dependence on opioids, all developed in association with the children leaving for college.

Here are some questions for you to consider. What was the nature of the mother's medical illness? Was it improperly diagnosed and treated? Was it instrumental in causing her psychiatric comorbidity? Could the indiscriminate use of barbiturates alone explain the mother's general deterioration? Among diagnoses considered for the mother's deterioration were major depressive disorder with psychotic features and a medical disorder affecting her brain such as tumor. Nothing was found using neuroimaging. Some of her symptoms are consistent with post-polio syndrome, a condition that often leads to weakness and fatigue and may be correlated with depressive disorder. Heavy metal toxicity (accounting for GI distress including abdominal pain and/or altered mental status) should also be ruled out. External stresses include children leaving for school and conflict with husband.

This case has moved from being reasonably straightforward to highly complicated, hardly solvable due to medical-psychiatric-social comorbidity. It all became "too much" for the patient. In the end, she committed suicide. And she did this in the most hideous way, by hanging herself. Supporting her decision to end her life, she claimed that her husband was having an affair. All we can do is speculate about the veracity of her reasoning. Whether it was based on fact or delusional?

This case illustrates the intersection of suspected systemic medical illness (never confirmed), dysfunctional family dynamics (patient and husband), disruptive events (sons leaving for college), and improper medical management, as well as patient susceptibility (patient's addictive vulnerability). The next case, Ben, in which depressive disorder was also prominent was entirely different. In that one, the patient presented with depressive disorder that was not well understood by his psychiatrist and was associated with "existential dreariness" (a neologism proposed by SAF). Tying the two cases together is suicide. The first patient did commit suicide, while the second patient barely escaped that end.

Case 2, Ben
Ben had everything to live for. He could not have been more successful as a computer programmer. When I first met him, he was 42-years-old, the father of twin girls. His wife was in a related profession. She was quite popular as an events coordinator and happy with her work. Not a bad profile except for one thing. Ben was morbidly depressed. While well-known for his work, he neither considered himself successful nor satisfied. To judge how odd this presentation was, witness the fact that Ben had been selected as the keynote speaker for the major meeting of his high-profile professional group.

Only a week after successfully delivering his talk (for which Ben did not need to extensively prepare), Ben began to develop suicidal thoughts and disappeared from his family for two weeks, hardly eating or talking. He lost interest in his work and did little more than ruminate about his perceived deficiencies and failures. Since none of these opinions was shared by others and he was not delusional, we are left with the diagnosis of severe major depressive disorder accompanied by suicidality.

Nurture

What is primarily at work here? Nature or nurture, biologically based depressive disorder, or depressive disorder based on experience such as trauma or emotional depravation in early life? What does a clinician risk when he or she approaches a case from a perspective that conflicts with the proper diagnostic designation of a patient's condition? To make this distinction, you probably need to know more. Ben had been raised in rural Australia in a poor family. His father was a salesman. Both parents were "emotionally unreachable." After secondary school, he enrolled in a publicly funded art college, but dropped out after a year, precipitously moving to England. Previously, he and the youthful band he organized had become widely known in Australia, and this experience qualified him to be hired by a well-known designer of record album covers after his arrival in England. Framing all this activity was Ben's brilliance as an artist and his musical accomplishments.

The picture is one of remarkable intellectual and artistic talent in the context of emotional poverty. When Ben finally left Australia, he was starkly alone. He maintained minimal contact with his parents and friends. He did not know where he was going, impetuously picking a destination, creating his future as he went along.

Ben's willingness to cooperate in his own recovery was impressive, but his lack of comprehension about the human elements missing from his professionally impressive life was profound. His marriage was unsatisfying and his relationship with his children distant. On reflection, it became clear that he had never experienced a committed human relationship, even though he could understand that these existed. In addition to cooperating with his psychiatrist's treatment recommendations (which included medication, electroconvulsive therapy (ECT), and repetitive transcranial magnetic stimulation (rTMS)), he needed to embrace new, in-depth, committed ways of being with others.

Nature: Ben's Biology

Move to the nature side. Given the depth of his depressive disorder, it was hard to imagine treating Ben without medication. Ben went through several cycles of medications. See Table 23.1 for breakdown: Side effects from lithium carbonate (doses adjusted according to regular blood levels) caused him to discontinue it. Several other medications were tried including venlafaxine extended release 37.5 mg daily as the starting dose (massive weight gain, somnolence, swollen joints), and citalopram 20 mg daily (insomnia, increased anxiety). Neither doxepin nor mirtazapine (starting dose 15 mg bedtime and then building to 30 mg bedtime) combined with small doses of lorazepam 1 mg was consistently helpful for sleep. Trazodone (50 mg bedtime) did help him sleep but produced "crazy dreams." Later, zolpidem (5 mg bedtime, increased to 10 mg bedtime) was introduced for sleep. A low dose of quetiapine 50 mg bedtime (for sleep) produced headaches and tremors.

Table 23.1 Ben's treatments in tabular form (medication changes during treatment not recorded)	Lithium carbonate (regular blood samples obtained for regulation)
	Doxepin 300 mg
	Venlafaxine XR 225 mg
	Citalopram 20 mg
	Lorazepam 1 mg, repeat x1 as needed
	Mirtazapine 15 mg
	Trazodone 50–100 mg
	Aripiprazole 20 mg
	Dextroamphetamine 10 mg as needed
	Bupropion XL 300 mg

Diazepam (5–10 mg 1×/day) kept him calm for most of the day but interfered with the clarity of his thinking at work. Aripiprazole (10 mg/day for anxiety) led to a 30-pound weight gain over 12 months. Dextroamphetamine 5 mg up to three times a day was used to combat "fogginess." Lamotrigine 300 mg daily was conditionally successful for mood stabilization, but Ben developed a rash and could not continue using it after 6 months. Bupropion 300 mg/day was tried for a short period but was "too simulating". After several years, Ben (thoughtfully) began to request that medications be reduced. He was cooperative and generally clear thinking throughout, often directing his own treatment by deciding when to cut back and when a new medication was needed.

Certainly, medication was conditionally helpful. But to what extent? Ben was able again to work but remained uninspired. He felt "bland" and "irritated" at having to work in a design firm where artistic values were superseded by business goals, making money, and competing on the job market the leading values. One possibility is that the medications he was using helped to regulate his mood but interfered with his capacity for excitement and creativity.

Ben eventually and uncomfortably revealed that he had a secret. One day during year 3 of treatment, Ben received a surprise phone call. It was from his estranged son, the product of a careless love affair when Ben was in his early 20s. His life from the time of the baby's birth had been a cover-up. His son, Ben, 25 at the time of this call wanted to see his father for the first time. This was not good news for Ben's already struggling marriage. Part of Ben's despair was attributed by him to this unsatisfactory marriage, a union lacking shared values and intellectual compatibility.

Back to the nature vs. nurture dichotomy before speculating about appropriate treatment. Let us assemble the building blocks first: extraordinary professional success significantly built on talent versus little meaningful connection to parents, abandonment of his out-of-wedlock son, an unsuccessful marriage distinguished by personal disconnection, and an equivocal relationship with twin daughters.

Progress. Taken all together, the descriptively most accurate summary of Ben's state of mind was that he was "*unhappy*." His despondency had become all encompassing, paralytic. There were an assortment of specific problems ranging from an abandoned son to marital dissatisfaction. Any of these issues could have been the basis for his despair. But none seemed to get to the heart of the matter. What seemed to matter most (according to Ben) was not feeling understood. Understanding Ben experientially, his isolation and his incompatibility with the values of his business partners are descriptive categories with no official place in psychiatric nosology. Recall that Ben was an unusually talented artist. His talent had led him to become famous in his field. To understand him, you would have to struggle to comprehend a personal world that was both powerful and very odd, lending to remarkable creativity. Medication or not, what seemed to be happening was that I was slowly coming to understand Ben in that way, allowing his experience to infiltrate me and become mine.

As we (Ben and SAF) worked together, several hard-to-explain developments occurred, all imperceptible and slow to progress. Ben resigned his high-profile but aesthetically unrewarding job; moved into the lead with his daughters' care, taking over much of it from his uninspired wife; and dedicated himself to his treatment in a new way. He also renewed his relationship with his out-of-wedlock son. At the same time, he became more realistic about what could be expected in his relationship with his wife.

I realize that I am implying that a special kind of interpersonal experience occurred in Ben's treatment with me and that this experience may have been a key to his recovery. This kind of claim is blasphemous in a professional world where science rules. "Science" means measurement, hard cold judgments about real-world phenomena and outcome. This statement allows me to return to "complexity," i.e., how things *really* work when you look at them closely, not simplify them. I cannot tell you *exactly* how Ben was able to heal in the context of our work and our dedication to his recovery. But I do have a good idea. Ben and I bonded in the most profound way. He could see that I really cared about him. Emphasis is on the word "really." Medication did seem to play an important part. Both Ben and I agree that children made a difference, providing a "second chance" for a meaningful life. However, more essentially, Ben was instrumental in creating for his daughters the kind of meaningful life he never had as a boy and participating in its richness. Associated with this process, he had the courage to leave his job and begin a new career as a photographer-author.

Subtle factors in the cases of the mother who took her own life and Ben emphasized *understanding*, a pressing desire that key figures in their lives truly understand the nature of their distress. Also, central in the "mother" case was children leaving home and a disconnected spouse. In Ben's case, the clinician, apart from providing medication, appreciated his unique talents and his intense need to have his perceptions validated. The practitioner also needed to understand how much the lack of this level of comprehension (and connection) had played in the development of Ben's despair.

In the following commentary by Ben, he articulated the experience described:

I do not have emotional investment in what I do. I feel lost when it comes to insisting on doing what I want to do. I'm often not sure of what I need. The result is that I almost always feel disappointed by other people: their inability to grasp nuance and read body language, moods, and emotions. What happens is that there is a weird impasse where I can't describe my state of mind to them. My business partner Rob and wife Carol do a very narrow set of things. We do not think the same way.

If I look back at the critical decisions I've made, they almost always involved someone who supported me. For music, they were primarily my mother and my friend Roger. The album we made was one of the most popular in the country but their encouragement was key. My success was the product of like minds working together. This kind of success is impossible to create if you do not have other people who believe in your ideas. You need at least one person around who believes in them and can enable them. My state of mind doesn't reflect emotional poverty but rather the absence of *comprehension by others*. It would help if Carol or Rob could say of my work, 'It's really cool.' My daughter Annabelle (who is wild and creative) has started to take that role for me.

Note that while Ben was reassured by Annabelle's comprehension and creative ability, it is nonetheless doubtful if anyone could truly understand the source of Ben's remarkable skill.

Problematic in Ben's case was his receiving the diagnosis major depressive disorder since it did not quite fit his experience. Ben described another, perhaps more potent, dimension of his psychological distress. He described it as being chronically unhappy insisting that the diagnosis "major depressive disorder" was inexact and didn't get to the "gut" issue. In the "Mother" example, Julia's assessment never included suicide. The ICD-10 depression scale had little to say about the patient's condition other than her being at least moderately depressed. Julia, the mother's primary care physician, recorded in her notes that the patient was "unhappy, discouraged, unable to progress" but little more.

Critical here is that patients' state of mind conformed solely neither to conventional diagnostic categories for depression (dysphoria, sadness, loss of interest) nor to its typical psychopathology. In contrast, the first patient, who I will call "Mother," might have preferred to describe herself as "abandoned with little else to live for." After all, what was left for her after her children left home and her husband defected? One could have categorized her state of mind as reflecting major depressive disorder, but she might not have agreed claiming that the diagnostician had not captured the essence of her despair. If someone had understood her on that level, her life might have been saved. Ben gave us the missing category for characterizing his mood, "not feeling understood." Clearly, this simple, more colloquial, category fit best for him.

The more conventional terms dysphoria and anhedonia may come close to describing their seriously impaired moods. But it is unlikely that either patient would agree that the label "major depression" accurately captures their unrelenting, existential suffering.

Formal Complexity Inventories; Complexity Assessment Tools

24

Introduction

Multimodal instruments designed to measure patient complexity are reviewed beginning with the Value-Based Intermed Complexity Assessment Grid (VB-IM-CAG), a gold standard for complexity assessment instruments. The VB-IM-CAG requires formal training to insure appropriate administration and scoring. Other related clinical instruments include (1) the Intermed Self-Assessment (IMSA) and (2) the Patient Centered Assessment Method (PCAM). These are abbreviated instruments and need less administration and scoring time than the VB-IM-CAG. They are also likely to be less dependable for clinical purposes. Finally, a new screening instrument for patient complexity is being developed by our group at the University of Minnesota and is intended for use together with the VB-IM-CAG.

In this chapter, we review abbreviated complexity assessment tools. These tools may range from screening instruments, typically consisting of a short list of questions for selecting candidates for participation in a research study, to more extensive self-assessment inventories, and those that are examiner-administered. At present, these time-saving instruments have not been adopted widely for incorporation into clinical programs for treating complex patients.

We know the discipline of medicine fundamentally rests on approximation. Statistics can zero in on the reliability of treatments. Ask a friend or relative how satisfied they were with a particular medical treatment. You are likely to find many who experienced initial delight when the result was what they had hoped for and may even believe they had been promised, but were abjectly disappointed when the initial "promise" didn't hold up. Shoulder surgery is a good example with hope dominant at first and pain with limitation so often resulting within a few years. Medical conditions tend not to stay static, with disease progression more the rule than the exception. Add new comorbid diseases that complicate diagnosis and treatment.

Complexity Profiling Inventories (Tools)

The Intermed Complexity Assessment Grid (IM-CAG) and its (almost identical) successor, the Value-Based Integrated Case Management Complexity Assessment Grid (from this point abbreviated "VB"), each yields a grid consisting of clinical items distributed across four clinical domains and rated in three time periods (historical, current state, "vulnerability" (prognosis)). Each complexity item ("anchor point") is constituted of two questions and responses that are rated by an examiner for medical urgency on a four-point scale. Each clinical item (anchor point) is connected in a computer program with a description and several goals and actions useful in addressing the problem at hand. The result is a color-coded profile that is intended for use in developing a treatment plan.

The VB-IM-CAG takes at least 45 minutes for an examiner (in our clinics, often a case manager) to administer. The administrator's job includes taking careful notes and placing findings on several scales to track the patient's progress. While this is an admirable endeavor, allowing for careful tracking, it is time-consuming and, in that way, may often be impractical. Consequently, Intermed-based abbreviated complexly tools have been developed that are intended either to substitute for the VB-IM-CAG (hereafter abbreviated as the "VB") or to screen for those patients whose presentation make them appropriate candidates to receive the VB.

Abbreviated Complexity Inventories

Significant effort has been made to create a practical alternative to the VB. The Intermed Self-Assessment (IMSA), a self-assessment inventory that follows the sequence of the VB-IM-CAG, was developed for this purpose. It is a 21-item self-assessment screen which was validated in 2017 in Europe in six centers in five European countries and was administered to a total of 850 patients [1]. It has the disadvantage of requiring somewhat complex scoring and requiring at least 15 minutes for administration (far less than the VB but still not cost-effective when used with large populations). The IMSA was additionally validated by our group with 110 HIV-positive patients in San Francisco and will be reported in the forthcoming publication, "The Validity of the INTERMED Self-Assessment Questionnaire in HIV-Infected Patients in the USA."

The Patient Centered Assessment Method (PCAM) [2] is a relatively brief examiner-administered assessment. It was developed at the University of Minnesota, Department of Family Medicine, and includes 12 categories across four dimensions (health and well-being, social environment, health literacy and communication, service coordination). It is rated on a four-point scale based on the urgency of required care. PCAM was validated in a preventative screening program in Scotland. This mixed-methods prospective cohort study was developed to establish its ability to identify mental health needs, and external validity for integrating the PCAM into existing health checks. Two studies are described: (1) a mixed-methods prospective cohort study of the implementation of the PCAM in primary care clinics and (2) a qualitative exploratory study that evaluated the value of the PCAM in a complex patient population.

Our research group at the University of Minnesota is developing a screening instrument likely consisting of 8–12 questions for initially selecting complex patients whose health issues should be prioritized. This project is being done in collaboration with colleagues at the University of Minnesota and includes Roger Kathol, MD, internal medicine and psychiatry in Minnesota, and Luke Rothermel, MD, an oncological surgeon in Cleveland, Ohio. The purpose of the screener is to identify complex patients who as an initial step in their evaluation require the VB to characterize and provide guidance for treating their clinical condition.

Summary

In addition to the two detailed complexity assessments, the interviewer-rated VB and the almost identical IM-CAG, we also have two validated, abbreviated assessment tools, the IMSA and PCAM. Our new, brief, complexity screening tool is under development.

The IMSA and PCAM have been created and validated in studies with adequate statistical power. However, neither instrument has been adopted for general use in part presumably because their clinical applicability has not been satisfactorily demonstrated. Problems besetting these abbreviated assessment instruments include the following. The clinical meaning of an elevated "complexity score" using each of these tools may not yet be clear or even useful to clinicians over a range of complex cases. What exactly does an elevated complexity score suggest about the patient's prognosis or workability using standard medical and interpersonal treatment techniques?

For example, a patient not only has poorly controlled diabetes mellitus but also is homeless. Finding food that is even marginally healthy is a challenge for this patient. The assessment and treatment challenges may be quite different for this patient than for a financially stable diabetic. What "workability" classification is most appropriate for this patient? We are not dealing with typical medical comorbidity; the health issues here exist in two separate dimensions. We are still left with the challenge of rating patients' severely compromised health situations where "health" includes social, emotional, and financial well-being.

To illustrate our dilemma, think of any medical condition. In this case, we select hypertension. Granted that while hypertension can ultimately be life-threatening, it is almost always initially "silent" and tends to damage the body progressively. Add that while in the military, your patient contracted syphilis. He paid little attention to this condition and in his last visit to the VA hospital, he was told that he now has "tertiary syphilis," and his kidneys were affected. There is certainly a lot to think about here. But wait. He has another pressing problem. His wife has recently been acting strangely, not coming home at the usual time at night. She has had a "mild" alcohol problem for years and had taken steps to fight it. But at about the time your patient began to notice his wife's tardiness, he also again began to smell alcohol on her breath in the evenings. The hooker here is social. How do you factor this interpersonal situation into your complexity equation?

Currently, the VB is the gold standard for profiling the health status of complex patients/cases like this one; the complexity screener we are developing (with the potential of being used in conjunction with the VB) could prove quite useful for initially spotting these patients. Our screener will be based on categories selected from the PCAM, IMSA, and an additional list of items selected by seasoned clinicians. If we are successful, we will be able to identify and set up ratings for clinical categories that have cross-dimensional relevance.

A complexity assessment tool should have at least the following characteristics:

- Diverse clinical items making a significant contribution to the psychological, personal (social), and physical (biological) health of the complex patients at issue
- The domains and time periods represented in the study
- Demographic categories relevant to the current study

Other Projects with Which We Have Been Involved that Address Clinical Complexity

The Silver Project for the assessment and treatment of HIV was conducted at the University of California, San Francisco 360: The Positive Care Center. The objective of this project was to create a "new integrated clinical and service models and protocols for persons 50 years of age and older in an HIV/HCV patient-centered medical home." Findings have not yet been published. For this project, each patient was administered an extensive health inventory, the VACS (Veterans Aging Cohort Study) Index. The VACS Index creates a score by summing pre-assigned points for age, CD4 count, HIV-1 RNA (routinely monitored indicators of HIV disease), and general indicators of organ system injury. Subjects contribute blood samples to determine the status of their HIV infection. Added are several screening tools including the Montreal Cognitive Assessment (MoCA). The VACS Index provides a measure of the health status of this group of complex medically and socially compromised patients and includes variables not included in the IMSA or PCAM. The VACS Index discriminates HIV-related risk of mortality more effectively than an index restricted to CD4 count, HIV-1 RNA, and age, especially among those with undetectable HIV-1 RNA levels. Our goal in this not yet completed study is to determine whether adding the IMSA to evaluate the level of complexity of our patients was helpful in identifying which patients required greater than usual care. We were able to carry out this study for only 1 year. Preliminary results supported the Silver Project screening as useful for categorizing these complex patients. Unfortunately, funding for this project has not been renewed. We are including it here since it is an example of a nicely designed study that considered multiple clinical categories across disparate dimensions. It illustrates the difficulty of conducting such a study over time.

The Challenge of Doing Research on Clinically Complex Cases

The challenge of doing research on clinically complex subjects can be summarized as "mixing apples and oranges." Try to wrap your brain around the following. You have three children: Carley, Pete, and Diane. Carley is 43-years-old, Pete 35, and Diane 21. As with all children, they have similarities and differences in part based on their genetics. You are looking for correlated categories (variables) that accommodate their similarities and differences. You need to know how to represent this situation according to traits. The following descriptions were supplied by family members. Carley is "cerebral" and thinks deeply, Pete is incisive and practical, and Diane is frivolous but, according to her mother, has a "great attitude about life believing that whatever else, it should be fun." You want to know about the common features of their personalities. Can these different "personality types" be joined into a meaningful unity? In this case, a consensus is needed to provide guidance about how to structure their roles in administering a family trust? What traits do these siblings have in common and how much disparity (variance) is there among them and what is the nature of the disparity?

It is OK to feel stymied as you consider this problem. In complex clinical work, you are not delivered problems in neat packages, and you do have to look for ways to encompass real-life similarities and differences to get a useful synthesis of the situation. For the record, the three human subjects under consideration do have commonalities. While not immediately apparent, these common areas may be more important personally to their collective lives than their differences. Carley provides the insight, Pete the practical solutions, and Diane the wisdom. But how can this situation be expressed numerically incorporating the contributions of each person to a consensus about how to manage the family trust?

Recapitulating

By this point, it must be clear that if you have only statistically validated, evidence-based practice guidelines, you are likely to have a gutless product, "mostly bones and little flesh." The value of idiographic renderings, clinical *descriptions* that include details that nomothetic depictions, cannot and should not be underestimated. Clinical situations up close are complicated. The cliché "the real person" is the true target for clinical representation. What else?

References

1. van Reedt Dortland AKB, Peters LL, Boenink AD, Smit JH, Slaets JPJ, Hoogendoorn AW, et al. Assessment of biopsychosocial complexity and health care needs: measurement properties of the INTERMED self-assessment version. Psychosom Med. 2017;79(4):485–92. https://doi.org/10.1097/psy.0000000000000446.
2. Maxwell M, Hibberd C, Aitchison P, Calveley E, Pratt R, Dougall N, et al. The Patient Centred Assessment Method for improving nurse-led biopsychosocial assessment of patients with long-term conditions: a feasibility RCT. Southampton: NIHR Journals Library; 2018.

Further Reading, PCAM Complexity Tool

Maxwell M, Hibberd C, Pratt R, Cameron I, Mercer S. Development and initial validation of the Minnesota Edinburgh Complexity Assessment Method (MECAM) for use within the keep well health check; 2011.

Pratt R, Hibberd C, Cameron I, Maxwell M. The Patient Centered Assessment Method (PCAM): integrating the social dimensions of health into primary care. J Comorb. 2015;5:110.

Yoshida S, Matsushima M, Wakabayashi H, et al. Validity and reliability of the Patient Centered Assessment Method for patient complexity and relationship with hospital length of stay: a prospective cohort study. BMJ Open. 2017;7:e016175.

Case Detail Presented in Narrative Form Versus Categorical Assessments, What Is Lost? What Is Retained?

25

Introduction

The use of heuristics is efficient for summarizing a clinical situation (a case). However, by reducing details the use of heuristics is likely to subtract from an accurate (detailed, in-depth) understanding of the patient.

Clinical work relies on heuristics to conveniently organize and summarize data. The living, breathing, suffering patient, however, tends to get lost in heuristic shorthand. In this chapter, we compare case description and heuristics as different approaches for representing the patient, to see what is gained or lost with each.

Both types of case information are likely to be relevant clinically: the former to summarize and categorize significant variables and the latter for describing the "whole patient," the human being to be evaluated and treated. The information conveyed may be quite different and lead to different treatment strategies. Someone with a high score on the PHQ-9 or the Hamilton Depression Scale may feel depressed, be unable to sleep, and behave lethargically at work and in social situations. However, that person may complain of qualitatively different symptoms than someone who presents for "depression" and describes suicidal ideation, preoccupation with the feeling that he or she is a failure, has lost social effectiveness, or is experiencing "emptiness" after the death of a spouse.

Clinical illustrations: Ben (2) and Thomas

These contrasting presentations can lead to different treatment strategies. The result of screening for depression may help decide which medication to prescribe. In that case, symptoms may be the deciding factor but not the description of the personal distress the subject is experiencing.

Here Is a Comparison

Categorical: DSM-5 Criteria for Major Depressive Disorder

Have you experienced five or more symptoms during the same 2-week period with at least one of the following (1) depressed mood or (2) loss of interest or pleasure? Select from the following edited list of symptoms (Table 25.1):

Table 25.1 DSM-5 criteria for major depressive disorder

To receive a diagnosis of major depressive disorder, five of these symptoms need to be present within the same 2-week period.

1. Depressed mood most of the day, nearly every day

2. Markedly diminished interest or pleasure in all, or almost all, activities most of the day, nearly every day

3. Significant weight loss when not dieting or weight gain or decrease or increase in appetite nearly every day

4. A slowing down of thought and a reduction of physical movement (observable by others, not merely subjective feelings of restlessness or being slowed down)

5. Fatigue or loss of energy nearly every day

6. Feelings of worthlessness or excessive or inappropriate guilt nearly every day

7. Diminished ability to think or concentrate, or indecisiveness, nearly every day

8. Recurrent thoughts of death, recurrent suicidal ideation without a specific plan, or a suicide attempt or a specific plan for committing suicide

Clinical Presentation (Source: Narrative from Interviews with Patient)

Return to Ben, our depressed computer programmer with a stunning reputation for creativity. His despair had become all-encompassing, paralytic. To summarize what has already been said about Ben, there was an assortment of problems ranging from boredom with his work to an abandoned son who suddenly insinuated himself into Ben's life, and dissatisfaction with his marriage. Any of these issues, in addition to his biology, could have been the basis for his depressed mood. While each factor may have been pertinent, none of these explanations got to the heart of the matter. According to Ben, what bothered him most was chronically "not feeling understood." To feel understood, Ben required comprehension of his sense of personal isolation. Recall that Ben was unusually talented as a computer programmer. With his talent, he became well-known in his field. To understand him, you would have to struggle to comprehend a personal world that was at the same time intense, attractive (not just aesthetically but also in terms of his humanistic preferences), and structurally very odd, all lending to his remarkable creativity. Medication or not, what seemed to be happening therapeutically was that I was slowly coming to understand Ben, allowing his personal experience to infiltrate mine and become "shared."

Ben's mood and productivity vacillated. These experiences were too emotionally complicated for categorical labeling. They were in part based on Ben's remarkable reasoning capabilities as reflected in his powerful positive and negative emotions when with people. The smallest disruption in rapport, a discordant experience that might not be noticed by another person, could seriously impede his ability to work. Creating a book of diagrams without words sent him soaring into elation. As we worked together, several hard to explain developments occurred, all imperceptible. Ben resigned his high-profile but aesthetically unrewarding job, took over his daughters' care from his vapid wife, and dedicated himself to treatment in a new way. He also renewed his relationship with his out-of-wedlock son. Compare the detail incorporated in this description of Ben and his life to a categorical statement of his clinical status.

Assessment and Choice of Treatment: Thomas

The analysis above leads to the topic of treatment. Any clinician who thinks critically knows that most treatment choices are at least somewhat arbitrary. It does not matter how closely your patient fits the chosen DSM-5 (or ICD 11) diagnostic category or how much confidence you have in the system that assisted you in your selection of a treatment modality.

Consider Thomas, age 25. Using psychometric assessment, Thomas was labeled as having "high-functioning autism." In his case, his autism spectrum disorder diagnosis (DSM-5 299.00) was combined with major depressive disorder (DSM-5 296.20). He was prescribed sertraline 50 mg/day, and after a year, since his depressive disorder seemed unrelenting and did not respond to increased medication, he received a series of ECT treatments. He experienced some relief from his depressive disorder, but not much. The situation had become dire once Thomas began struggling to keep suicidal thoughts out of his mind. Thomas' father had been a brilliant scientist and Thomas harbored aspirations of having a similar career. Thomas kept telling his psychiatrist he believed that his depressive disorder "clearly had a biological component" but that he was also convinced that "the psychological contribution was significant." This situation remained symptomatically static for 2 years during his late teens. Relief only came after Thomas was admitted to college to study biology. The experience that jolted him ahead was organic chemistry. Most of the other students struggled, but Thomas found organic chemistry "easy," so easy that he mastered the entire semester's assignments in a few weeks.

Thomas took to chemistry just like some people take to snowboarding. A year later, he was studying quantum mechanics and thermodynamics. He was not entirely free of depression, but according to him, his depression was "80%" better. In addition to psychotherapy, he had been tried with little success on an array of medications including aripiprazole 2 mg each morning and following that a tricyclic antidepressant, amitriptyline 50 mg a day. Was it the depression rating scale (HAM-D) and medication, or the clinical-interpersonal management that pierced this cycle? You choose. Our position is that they likely worked in concert. The clinical management with a psychiatrist who Thomas liked and respected was undoubtedly centrally implicated in his recovery. Also, Thomas' entry into a professional field in which he had considerable talent must have counted heavily.

Where to go from here? Thomas wanted to give up medication soon. He knew this was risky and might trigger a relapse. He felt he had come a long way and most importantly had gained what he believed was significant control over his current life and future.

Return to Complexity Assessment Tools

Return to our "Intermed" derived complexity assessment tools (the "VB," the IMSA, and the PCAM). Each of these assessments provides a number (a "complexity" rating) which combines the individual results from "anchor point" ratings in four domains: medical, psychological, social, and care delivery (availability of care for that patient). As noted above, the value of the complexity score obtained by the IMSA for making predictions about treatment efficacy over 3- and 6-month follow-up periods has been confirmed by both our group in San Francisco and in a 1998 study in Europe involving 850 participants in six different countries (Heiligenberg, M.). The complexity scores obtained using the IMSA can be used to decide whether a patient requires a definitive assessment using the full interviewer-rated VB-ICM-CAG (VB). The VB provides a clinical profile using rated anchor points and a narrative appraisal of the patient consisting of meticulously conducted interviews by the patient's clinician, often a case manager. Voila! We have moved past the strictly categorical (multiple choice) assessment to the inclusion of a narrative.

To be honest, there is nothing intuitive about how to include four dimensions, three time periods, and assorted assessment items in a single assessment. As you can imagine, putting all this information together in a way that is statistically valid has been more than a little challenging. A clinical opinion that excludes the social or the psychiatric dimensions, or a weighted measure of each contributing category is likely to be anemic, incomplete in essential ways not representing the human being that the patient is.

Limitations of Complexity Assessment Tools

26

Introduction

The Intermed Self-Assessment (IMSA) can be used to identify and measure (self-report) clinical complexity. This self-assessment instrument is easier to use and more time- and cost-efficient than the more fully elaborated VB-IM-CAG. Nevertheless, the IMSA may not be precise enough to be useful in many clinical situations. In this chapter, we recommend a two-step approach to complexity assessment consisting of (a) the screening instrument we are currently developing and validating and when indicated (b) the sequential administration by a trained examiner of the VB-IM-CAG.

The IMSA ("Intermed Self-Assessment") is an abbreviated complexity assessment tool. The IMSA consists of 21 questions that follow the structure of the VB-IM-CAG. Its advocates make claims about its ability to identify treatment requirements in complex clinical situations. The IMSA is one of the two abbreviated complexity assessment tools of which we are aware, the other being the PCAM (Patient Centered Assessment Method). The IMSA is useful for rating patients according to their "level" of complexity, a designation that includes data from four and potentially five clinical domains (biological, psychological, social, health care, and vulnerability).

Our IMSA (Intermed Self-Assessment) validation project at the University of California San Francisco (UCSF) was based on a well thought out research plan. There were about 110 participants, each of whom received an extensive survey consisting of questions in four different dimensions, medical, psychiatric, social, and care delivery (level of care received), and cutting across three time dimensions (past, current, prognosis). Statistical analysis found that this abbreviated complexity assessment tool could predict numbers of emergency room visits, hospital admissions, outpatient visits, and diagnostic exams with reasonable accuracy. Subjects were again interviewed at 6 and 12 months. The instrument was validated at six European institutions in five different countries, with a total of 850 patients (van Reedt Dortland et al., 2017). During

S. A. Frankel et al., *Complexity in Health Care*,
https://doi.org/10.1007/978-3-031-14949-8_26

its 4-year duration, this project was well executed by veteran researchers. However, oddly (!), the resulting instrument has hardly ever used for clinical purposes. Presumably, it was regarded as impractical by clinicians. It takes only 10–20 minutes to administer and is a self-assessment instrument requiring no examiner. The most labor-intensive aspect of using this tool is scoring the 20 items comprising the survey. With a bit more work by a programmer, the instrument could be computer-scored. The answer to this puzzle ironically seems to be that the IMSA is not capable of yielding *useful* enough information. The predictions have too many associated "what ifs." What if the patient cannot find transportation to the ER, does not have a PCP, and has several comorbid conditions so that the complexity that the test identifies reflects a condition that is too amorphous for the test to be immediately useful?

Feedback from clinicians about the utility of this painstakingly developed measure suggests that the subject matter, clinical complexity, is hardly amenable to categorical assessment. There are so many subcategories at issue, many of which require clinician and/or patient appraisal (both opinions are subjective). How to rate the patient's pain? Its intensity as contrasted to previous manifestation when it was readily controllable with an NSAID seems so much greater. The patient says that the pain is "excruciating." Should we include in our appraisal the possible significance of his argument with his son earlier that week? It almost led to blows.

The IMSA is elegant, but can it be useful? If not, are there no tools that can usefully direct us through clinically complex situations such as this one? Our opinion is that complexity assessments might better be done in two parts. The first step would consist of administering a screener designed to identify clinically complex situations requiring skilled intervention by a clinician who can administer and score the VB. The second step would be administration and scoring of the VB by a skilled clinician such as a case manager. That person rates the severity and character of the patient's complaints, invokes other assessment measures if needed, and conducts an extensive clinical interview with the patient. This design is in fact the one we use for identifying and evaluating clinically complex situations requiring clinician intervention.

Part XI

Remaining Groups of Variables

[Part Introduction: The requirement for well-conceived clinical work may be anything but straightforward. Many clinical variables are elusive ("#2" variables) and difficult to efficiently target with a conventional course of treatment. In this part, we consider this elusive component of clinical work, its contribution to the clinical situation, and what is lost when these contributions are minimized by clinicians. These come under the heading of "#2" and "#3" variables (which will be defined later in the book). These clinical situations may be hard to both characterize and target with treatment. Precision medicine is increasingly being developed to address these highly specific needs. These developments are generally beyond the scope of this book but should be appreciated if one wants to understand that these precision techniques exist and to have a full appreciation of the stuff out of which clinical situations are made. Examples include the use of nanoengineered enzymes to bind to a tumor cell so that the body's natural cell degradation can eliminate those cells from the body. As a form of molecular medicine, targeted therapy may block the growth of cancer cells. Often the agents of targeted therapy are biopharmaceuticals. Biologic therapy is often synonymous with targeted therapy for cancer treatment.

The topic of highly complex, often elusive, clinical contributions is central to this book. When their contribution to clinical work is not appreciated the character and importance of that clinical situation is likely to be underestimated or overestimated.]

Elusive Variables ("#2" Variables), Anxiety, Mood, Excitement (Sexual and Otherwise), Motivation, and Judgment

27

Introduction

The focus of this chapter is on "#2" (elusive) variables, i.e., variables that are not discrete (amorphous) and may be hard to define with precision. The exemplar in this chapter is that of a patient with a possible diagnosis of Crohn's disease. If the clinician centers his/her attention only on the most common symptoms of Crohn's disease, e.g., diarrhea or malaise, he or she may fail to consider less common symptoms. Moreover, the clinician may miss competing explanations for symptoms such as those related to side effects of medication.

Diseases may be diffuse in their manifestations, affecting multiple organs and/or organ systems often in nonspecific ways. Presenting symptoms may include side effects of medication which mimic manifestations of the disease itself. Ben's Crohn's disease is used for illustration.

Clinical Illustration: Ben

What clinical factors fall outside the scope of conventional variables and into hard to define, measure, and track areas of clinical activity? So far, we have seized on definable clinical entities ("#1" variables). But, what about factors that are hard to visualize and define or are simply elusive? There is no scarcity of these in clinical work. Attitude, motivation, and interpersonal connection are some of these categories, all heavy with subjectivity. Most medical literature strives to be clear when naming and describing disease entities. The elusive parts for a medical picture are often in the "rule outs."

Clinical illustration: Ben—Crohn's disease (3)

With Ben, the rule outs started with a medical condition that was omitted from the initial description of his condition, rule out Crohn's disease. Crohn's disease is a chronic inflammatory bowel disease. Ben had occasional flare-ups resulting in periods of pain and disablement. Honestly, it was hard to tell whether the problem for Ben was Crohn's disease, an anxiety disorder, and/or side effects from infliximab, the immunosuppressive agent to control painful and destructive flare-ups. How to know which to choose?

Here is where the confusion begins. Side effects of infliximab include abdominal pain, back pain, nausea, and diarrhea. Wait. Are not these symptoms of Crohn's itself?

Look at a list of potential side effects for this medication, or equally a detailed list of manifestations of the disease itself with prevalence data from meta-analyses [1] (from UpToDate). Crohn's disease is an immune-mediated inflammatory disease that can affect any portion of the intestinal tract from the mouth to the anus. It can be associated with the following (Table 27.1):

Table 27.1 Potential side effects for infliximab

Potential side effects for infliximab:
Abdominal pain—44%
Diarrhea—39%
Weight loss—23%
Rectal bleeding—21%
Fever—14%
Fatigue—9%
Perianal disease—8%
Poor growth—7%
Joint pain—7%
Vomiting—7%
Nausea—6%
Mouth sores—3%
Treatment with infliximab is commonly associated with:
• Stomach and chest pain
• Chills
• Cough, runny nose, sneezing
• Respiratory infections, such as sinus infections and sore throat
• Dizziness or fainting
• Fatigue or weakness
• Difficulty breathing (shortness of breath)

Table 27.1 (continued)

- Tightness in the chest
- Fever
- Flushed face
- Headache
- Hives
- Muscle pain
- Nausea
- Low blood pressure or high blood pressure
- Rash or itching

Table 27.2 Additional relevant diagnostic tests

Included are:
• Diagnostic tests for serum iron; calcium; magnesium; folate; vitamins A, E, and B12; and zinc
• Tissue biopsy
• Imaging: colonoscopy and sigmoidoscopy
• Blood tests including CBC with differential count, platelets, ESR, C-reactive protein, serum total protein, and albumin; ALT, AST, SGTP (to assess for hepatobiliary disease, including primary sclerosing cholangitis)
• Stool tests: guaiac, stool for leukocytes, calprotectin; stool bacterial culture, smears for ova and parasite, *C. difficile* toxin assay
• Tuberculosis screening (tuberculin skin test)
• Titers for varicella and measles; HBV serologies
• Urinalysis

Ben had intermittent bouts of diarrhea, mild to moderate stomach pains on most days. He often felt nauseated. His joints ached. There is little information suggesting local causes for these joint pains including mechanical overload and repetitive movements. Listing these mostly nondescript symptoms in a patient workup can be distracting taking the clinician's attention away from more blatant central manifestations and causes. To confirm and enlarge upon specific diagnostic tests may help but may not be definitive (Table 27.2).

It can be helpful to zero in on a diagnosis through additional laboratory testing, in this case to further characterize type of inflammatory bowel disease. Additional studies for Ben might include:

- P-ANCA, ASCA
- Investigating other causes of diarrhea: lactose/glucose hydrogen breath test for lactose intolerance/bacterial overgrowth, 72-h fecal fat quantitation, and stool alpha-1-antitrypsin (Table 27.3)

Table 27.3 Additional radiographic studies for small bowel disease

For additional radiographic studies for localization of small bowel disease, the following might be tried:
• Magnetic resonance elastography
• UGI/small bowel follow through
• Abdominal CT with oral contrast
• Additional tests as indicated, depending upon clinical findings: bone age, abdominal plain films, fistulogram, ultrasound, or HMPAO leukocyte scan (labeled white blood cell scan)

Endoscopic studies:

- Colonoscopy (including ileoscopy) with biopsies
- Upper endoscopy with biopsies

In summary, symptoms reflecting Crohn's disease are often nonspecific. The origin may remain obscure especially when the symptoms represent autoimmune manifestations or a generalized affliction as is the case with "medically unexplained symptoms (MUS)" including chronic fatigue syndrome (myalgic encephalomyelitis). Laboratory tests may help identify the type of GI disease, but their specificity may not be adequate to fully rule out other etiologies. Not only is Crohn's a chronic condition but symptom elusiveness may add considerably to the challenge of diagnosing and treating it.

Emphasized here is uncertainty and nuance. This is the complexity of medical complexity emphasizing the uncertain and/or unknown. It is tempting to highlight clear-cut and bothersome symptoms such as diarrhea with a Crohn's disease pattern for focus, but the risk is of missing core pathology by not paying attention to less discrete symptoms.

Reference

1. Peppercorn MA, Kane SV. Crohn disease (beyond the basics). Official reprint from UpToDate® © 2022 UpToDate, Inc. 2022.

Anxiety, Mood, Excitement (Sexual and Otherwise), Motivation, and Judgment

Introduction

Nebulous, difficult to define and measure, and fluctuating are some of the characteristics of "#2" variables. Theoretical and operational definitions of these variables can be hard to establish. Nonetheless, "#2" variables are prominent features of most clinical situations. Key ideas about the nature and importance of such variables are discussed in this chapter.

The requirement for well-conceived clinical work may be anything but straightforward. Many clinical variables are elusive ("#2" variables) and difficult to efficiently target with a conventional course of treatment or even to name with precision. In this chapter, we consider this elusive component of clinical work, its contribution to the clinical situation, and what is lost when these inexact contributions are minimized by clinicians.

"#2" Variables

In this chapter, we will bring to life "#2" clinical variables, a range of elusive, often deemphasized clinical factors that are a major focus of this book. Start with anxiety. What is anxiety? Initially, it is one of those abstract "constructs" that needs to be explicated using more concrete observables. How can you define and measure anxiety? For a definition leading to concrete representations, you can use self-report data, behavioral measures such as interference with thinking or with structured activities, physiological criteria such as skin conductance, or decreased alpha and increased beta brain waves on EEG. People suffering from anxiety may have catastrophic expectations, be unable to concentrate, in some instances become marginally or temporarily delusional, or limit their thinking and activities to block

© The Author(s), under exclusive license to Springer Nature Switzerland AG 2023
S. A. Frankel et al., *Complexity in Health Care*,
https://doi.org/10.1007/978-3-031-14949-8_28

unwanted thoughts and feelings. But what is anxiety, and how to explain its lack of shape and its elusiveness despite its centrality in human experience? Apart from its consequences, it is more than a little hard to measure. Like so many other clinical-behavioral phenomena, measurement can best be done indirectly, i.e., through its consequences.

Mood, excitement (sexual and otherwise), motivation, and judgment are concepts that are equally difficult to define and measure. "Clinical experience" and "clinical judgment," both heavily subjective concepts (existing in the mind of the subject), not only count in clinical work, but they may even dominate clinical activity. These are elusive, at times subtle, but often potent factors, coloring clinical activity and potentially affecting both patient and clinician. They have their bases in the mind and/or body of the patient, for example, pain and its nuances, mood and its spectrum, anxiety and its omnipresence, pleasure including love and sexual experience, the feelings associated with ambition, and the desire to focus and achieve.

Consider the following clarifications:

- Emotion: e.g., an emotional reaction does not simply represent a "subjective state" of mind. It is, of course, related to the development of describable phenomena called "feelings." Emotional experiences are elusive, resistant to sharp definition. The neurological, biochemical, and endocrine bases of emotions have been documented. But the feelings themselves cannot be tightly contained and defined [1].
- Judgment: a process which is specific and often incorporates an interpersonal component. Judgment almost always has an object, a focus. This focus may be a personal; practical, e.g., a decision; or in the field of medicine, treatment. Nonetheless, judgment is infused with subjectivity.
- Motivation: Motivation is a driver of personal productivity. But where does its energy come from and how is it sustained? We know that context matters a great deal for initiating and supporting motivation. In the presence of negative emotion (discouragement), motivation suffers.

All these hard-to-portray states of mind add nuance to experience. In that sense, these experiences can be thought of as poorly "bounded." Let's try "love." How often have you been impressed by how "alike" you think your feelings are to another person's, only to discover rifts, differences in emotion, incompatible beliefs, and/ or biases?

It is time to regroup. All these amorphous streams of "#2" variables flow into our usual, reasonably ordered world, potentially adding uncertainty to it. If you choose to work with one of our detailed case descriptions as opposed to a nomothetic simplification, do you not risk getting lost or bogged down? Wouldn't you do better to stay with the simplified version? However, go back to our cases and make note of the risk of getting it wrong if you oversimplify. What would Seth's case be like if we took his mother out of the picture? Or Omar's case without reference to his captivity? Can Herb's case be understood without including his hiding his symptoms from his wife and physician?

Reference

1. Ekman P. Emotions revealed: recognizing faces and feelings to improve communication and emotional life. New York, NY: Henry Holt; 2007.

Clinical Work with "#2" Variables

Introduction

This chapter is a continuation of the discussion of "#2" variables. These variables are contrasted to the more concrete and measurable "#1" variables. In this chapter, we further mention two elusive clinical variables, motivation and "making love."

Returning to the topic of "motivation," Martin, age 20, said he finally had become motivated to apply himself at school. He thought he would become a professional musician. He knew the date of each upcoming music concert in and around San Francisco. He could tell you all the details, including the dates and locations of each group's last five performances. It is impressive, a little like the encyclopedic knowledge of baseball statistics that the boys in my neighborhood were so good at reciting when I was a teenager. His psychotherapist says that she is not clear about how to motivate Martin. What part of his psyche needs to be engaged? (1) The incipient understanding that at age 20 he needs to be thinking of a vocation? (2) His capacity to act in his own behalf given his habituation and possible addiction to cannabis? (3) His dislike of regimentation, an attitude that has been with him since his mother proposed that he do his part in earning money for his upkeep?

It might be better if we knew exactly what we are targeting. So, even "motivation" with its implicit goals and "making love" with its physical connotations aren't very coherent concepts. They are slippery. It is handy and likely correct to use the word "subjective" to justify our lack of clear focus when we use phrases like "making love" or words like "motivation."

Clinical illustrations: Martin and his problem with motivation, and comment on the meaning of "making love"

S. A. Frankel et al., *Complexity in Health Care*,
https://doi.org/10.1007/978-3-031-14949-8_29

Clinical Precision Versus Approximation Through Statistics

What is the relationship between approximation and subjectivity? Mathematics (the science of numbers, quantities, space, and their operations) involves determining the exact results of quantitative postulations using arithmetic and its operations. It is the same with calculus, although that mathematical system describes change and progression on a point-by-point basis. Statistics is devoid of this kind of exactness. In contrast, the study of statistics deals with acceptable approximations: the probability that an event has or will occur.

So, even with statistics, we are cast back into a universe of approximations. It's not "making love" that is real and tangible. It is targeting part of that experience, magnifying its coordinates, and giving it a label. The final task is placing the concept into a context and confirming through consensus that something about the experience is "real" and useful.

Our topic now is subjectivity. Variables that may be difficult to pin down without operational definitions. There are (at least) two parallel sets of variables in complex clinical fields:

- **"#1" Variables.** Standard, definable, and generally clearly understood by others. These may be manifest as definitions or instructions, i.e., algorithms.
- **"#2" Variables.** Those that are characterized by their subjectivity and protean-like behavior. These variables tend to be amorphous, hard to define with precision, and elude containment, e.g., anxiety.

The inclusion and tracking of both categories of variables are fundamental to conceptualizing clinical complexity (its structure, evolution, and management). Much of the remaining portions of this book will be spent working through and utilizing this model, always keeping the presence and management of "#2" and "#3" variables in mind.

Detecting, Organizing, and Prioritizing "#2" Variables

30

Introduction

This chapter contains a further explication of "#2" variables along with comparisons and contrasts to "#1" variables. Interactions between variable types are illustrated.

Jess' behavior, discussed later in the chapter, illustrates the interaction of the plethora of often elusive "#2" variables. The matrix of clinical work is complicated and ever shifting with variables reinforcing and negating one another. Each "#2" variable we have described, associated with Juliana's situation to Ben's, has its own configuration associated with its use and meaning in everyday life.

It is interesting to note that "#2" variables are often more ubiquitous in clinical situations than "#1" variables. Each calls out in a very different "voice": Juliana's with crankiness, Omar's with surreptitiousness, Nafi's with romanticism, and Ben's with stubborn isolation. If all this is true, the fallacy of lumping variables such as these into categories (such as diagnostic categories) is underscored. Juliana, Omar, Nafi, and Ben were all depressed (a restricted diagnostic category). But meet them on the street and they may be as different as night and day. And they each exist within their own unique subjective cloud. In fact, getting them to talk together and agree about issues might be nearly impossible since they are so different from one another.

Return to what separates them. Each person has different "#1" concerns, Juliana her fortune and pride, Omar his safety, and Nafi his bland past. And all (as you would guess) exist in vastly different subjective "#2" clouds. Juliana's, her unrelenting sense she will be betrayed; Omar's, his distrust; Nafi's, his misplaced trust; and Ben's, his ever-present gloom.

Clinical illustration: Jess

S. A. Frankel et al., *Complexity in Health Care*, https://doi.org/10.1007/978-3-031-14949-8_30

Again, our task is to picture a profoundly disparate and complicated clinical field but with at least two main sets of variables, those that are familiar and definable and those that are elusive and resistant to definition and measurement. Each variable has a unique character, and each makes its own contribution to the overall clinical field. Clinical work in its complexity is rather like this. It consists of uncountable numbers of disparate elements. Medicine—as an example—is constituted of disease categories "#1", together with "#2" (elusive, largely subjective) elements referring to the character, manifestations, and consequences of the disease. All of these variables affect and potentially infect one another. "#3" variables will be added to our list of variables to provide depth.

To illustrate, picture each "#1" variable as having its own "mini-magnetic" field, each mini-field attracting and/or repelling. A large concentration of these mini-fields would have a greater magnetic effect on the entire situation than collections with fewer numbers of these fields. Then, imagine that each center (concentration) of magnetic influence generates a different color which is a function of its density. The configurations of magnetic influence and color patterns produced would be variegated and intriguing. The practical outcome (magnetic influence and color configurations) would be different for each cluster. Using vectors, we could add up the magnetic fields by strength and the colors by candela (a measure of luminosity). The outcome would be experienced as a composite, a mix of all elements.

Discussed "#2" variables from Chapter 28 were emotion (e.g., anxiety), judgment, and motivation. Of course, there are many more examples of "#2" variables. As noted, they tend to, but do not exclusively, fall within the realm of subjectivity. The Merriam Webster dictionary (2004) defines "emotion" as (1) the "affective aspect of consciousness, (2) a state of feeling, (3) a conscious mental reaction (such as anger or fear) subjectively experienced as feeling usually directed toward a specific object and typically accompanied by physiological and behavioral changes in the body." Note how many nuances and ramifications (each a variable within the clinical field) these definitions offer.

Steps in Experiencing and Expressing an Emotion

Here is an example of what happens when there is an experienced emotion (Table 30.1):

Clearly, unlike with "#1" variables, this experience is likely to be unfocused. It probably seems very real to the subject, but its essence is emotional and physiological. This phenomenon, let's call it "sadness," is momentarily unbounded. It can be experienced as more or less impactful. It can be isolated within the current clinical situation or dominate it. Nonetheless, in its minor forms, it often slips past the observer. In its more overt manifestation, it may be associated with a diagnosis, "major depressive disorder." But "depression" is an abstraction and when invoked

Table 30.1 Progression following an experienced emotion

1. "I feel sad"

2. There is monoamine release and/or suppression, as well as potentially an endocrine response

3. I find myself recalling other instances that have resulted in similar feelings, e.g., in this case perhaps post-traumatic in character

4. I respond by withdrawing or becoming vigilant. This response may occur in a split second or last longer

5. The emotion either builds or fades

6. Others may be enlisted to help

can be formalized as one of several subtypes of mood disorder, including major depression, persistent depressive disorder, bipolar disorder, seasonal affective disorder (sad), psychotic depression, peripartum (postpartum) depression, premenstrual dysphoric disorder (PMDD), 'situational' (reactive) depression.

"#2" Variables: Redefinition

Moving closer to a definition of "#2" variables, then, we might characterize them as (1) occupying clinical/personal/emotional "space"; (2) affecting outcome to an extent that may be unexpected; (3) being serpentine, unbounded, and/or ephemeral, i.e., intangible; and (4) resistant to measurement. With these characteristics, no wonder these variables are frequently bypassed, minimized, and/or treated carelessly in clinical writing. "#2" variables are pervasive. When they are neglected, the clinical situation is necessarily overly simplified and misrepresented.

Deconstruction of Jess' Dysphoria

We could use Jess, age 27, to illustrate. She had been adopted at birth to an abusive mother. Her professionally competent but emotionally limited father raised her following a divorce. Her saga consisted of multiple psychotherapist transfers and residential treatments. She became attached to a psychotherapist who remained the steady figure in her life despite Jess' repeated failures. Her course was always rocky (as happens often in unsuccessful adoptions) with multiple attempts to "get on the right track."

"#1" variables here are adoption at birth and her father's marriage to and divorce from Jess' first of two adoptive mothers. Included is Jess' need for attachment and initial willingness to bond to available nurturing figures. Then came father's marriage to a woman to whom Jess never attached and for whom Jess' remained a focus for hostility. Finally, there is Jess' powerful, yet inconsistent, bond to her psychotherapist. "#2" variables were related to Jess' chronic dissatisfaction and her incapacity to make heartfelt, secure attachments.

This situation has parallels to the "mini-magnetic field" model of clinical influence. Despite the potential for bonding with multiple attachment figures, each interpersonal situation successively breaks down for Jess. If this model is confusing to you, that's understandable since it is built on a structurally and emotionally unstable human template. If it sounds too abstract, however, it isn't. You could take the named situations in Jess' unfolding life and come up with a model that guides you in predicting each successive phase.

In the next chapter, we will tackle the chaotic world involving the coexistence and interaction of "#1" and "#2" variables. God forbid, we may get lost.

Creation of a New Model for Clinical Practice

31

Introduction

In this chapter, randomness (stochastic distributions of variables) is added as one of the potential characteristics of "#2" variables. The unexpected events involving two previously discussed patients, Nafi and Seth, illustrated the observation that seemingly random phenomena tend to become organized over time, albeit in ways and with outcomes that may be surprising. Complex physical phenomena involve many constituents, and may be influenced by numerous forces, and exhibit unexpected or emergent behavior. Often such complex systems include subordinate subsystems or are subsumed into a more general system that may or may not be dominant.

With the emphasis on complexity and randomness of clinical events, we enter a new world for clinical practice, one where events are not necessarily tightly organized or sequential. It seems like we have started to create a new model, a collection of factors leading to a modified clinical theory and practice. Its identity centers on the elusive, not fully defined variables that populate clinical interaction. What happens if these "#2" variables are left out or even minimized? In that case, we find ourselves in a universe that "lacks a human face." The clinical situation you erect isn't real. As a practitioner, you hardly have time or patience to include all or even most "#2" clinical variables in your thinking. But do you have a choice? How else can you maintain the "real" clinical situation in your thinking and recommendations?

Let us take a moment and return to a model that prominently includes "#2" variables. "#2" variables are not precisely formulated, lack stability and clear definition. Add randomness, i.e., a stochastic distribution of events.

Clinical Illustrations: Herb and Jess

© The Author(s), under exclusive license to Springer Nature Switzerland AG 2023
S. A. Frankel et al., *Complexity in Health Care*,
https://doi.org/10.1007/978-3-031-14949-8_31

Nonetheless, we know from physics that random situations do tend to organize, often in obscure ways. This restructuring presumably happens because of influential factors, analogous to our mini-magnetic fields (Chapter 30), embedded in a clinical situation.

Let's work backward. In analogy to random variables, we are struck by the absence of logical sequence in our clinical examples. Events don't necessarily follow in expected order. Why do I feel love when I have just been angry at my wife? The glue is in part an obscure factor described by human psychology, not objectivity or logic. The sequence might be bounded in conventional ways, i.e., your wife is still your wife, and you are loyal to her. However, it is possible that the end point of this sequence will be quite different than the one you imagined and will be based significantly on emotions and other intangible factors. Both "#1" and "#2" variables play important roles in this process.

We still need a better answer to the question of why muddy our thinking with so much detail? Why would any self-respecting physician wedded to economy of thinking and order adopt such a complex model? Movement toward standard use of algorithms and biologically based diagnoses and treatments argues against the utility of our complexity model. However, we are left with the question of whether there actually are acceptably accurate clinical models that are simpler and more straightforward than ours? We believe the answer is no! That is if one does not want to take "the life out of" clinical work by oversimplifying and excessively objectifying it.

Now Return to Jess

Jess' first adoptive mother abused her. She couldn't stand Jess' childish demands. She screamed at and hit Jess when Jess fussed. Her father was even-handed but distracted by his dental practice. He failed to shield Jess. He was caring but incapable of thinking psychologically. Her attachment to this adoptive mother was distorted and spotty. Her attachment to her father was strong but defective. The fact that he had married Jess' mother is a giveaway. The separation from her occurred when Jess was about 18 months old. Pay attention to "#2" variables: care, love, and attendant attachment. Especially recognize how elusive these concepts were in this case.

Jess' second adoptive mother was competitive for Jess' father's attention. She was convinced that she had a special ability to understand children. She was unaware of her animosity toward Jess. The result was for Jess to identify her as a mortal enemy. Alienating this mother and putting Jess' father in a difficult position, having to take sides.

The "#1" variables in this situation include Jess' age, her lack of attachment to her first adoptive mother, the abuse she had encountered up through 18 months of age, the hostile attachment to her second adoptive mother, and the father's incapacity to understand Jess' deeper needs. The "#2" variables included Jess' temperament and her innate intelligence which was strong according to cognitive testing and helped her to progressively understand the realities of her inadequate parenting situation. The "#2" variables shifted as Jess moved from her first adoptive mother to the second. Different forms of hostility and alienation evolved in interaction with successive sets of parents who could not understand her needs. Add sexual maturation which in part because of insecurity engendered her two adoptions became distorted into attention seeking (and anger when she was disappointed by boys who originally promised love and commitment but failed to carry through).

Everything here is partially random, propelled by forces that came up without anticipation. The outcome of this situation is partly fueled by "#1" variables, for example, in Jess' case, the probable outcome of an abusive situation between birth and 18 months of age and two ambivalently regarded adoptions. Added are the many "#2" factors at work here including the influence of Jess' age and her responses as events occurred, her temperament, and unpredictable parental behavior over time.

Random Clinical Phenomena and How It Organizes: Herb

So, how does random phenomena organize? Think of it clinically. Herb was hurting all over. He was intermittently febrile. There was blood mixed with his stool. But he also was embarrassed and scared. What would he do if his wife found out? How would his job and professional ambitions be affected? What is the organizing focus (or foci) here? It is not the disease itself. It is the disease adulterated with "#2" "stuff," i.e., emotions. It's the "stuff" which clinicians often prefer to overlook because it makes what we do seem chaotic, in fact "messy." No one really knows what to do with it.

But! Ironically, we all live with it, and no one is truly oblivious to it. Jess is always dismissive. Her therapist can't really penetrate her, find her "soul," and detect the principles that underlie her messy inner world. This is not meant to sound scientific because it isn't unless you dig deeply enough. I have a lovely collie dog (Sherpa) who seems to be aware of everything going on around him. Unlike Jess, he can keep it all pretty simple. A new smell gets isolated, so it is primary in his mind. If he hears another dog in the distance, he switches his attention but doesn't seem to forget the original scent.

This is our first clue to the organizing principles for randomness: follow your nose and your ears. The key is sorting it out, so you pay attention to one thing at a time. But, like my dog, you cannot lose sight of any part of the tapestry since each element is part of a whole. It is a little like the mini-magnetic field analogy from Chapter 30.

In statistics, you deal with multiple data points that organize into "curves" when you graph them. You estimate the values of new data points using regression analysis but the curves (even those that are "corrected") are at least somewhat arbitrary. In real life, we act according to formulas (algorithms) and use these to make decisions. But there is nothing sacred about our choices. They are in part subjective.

Let's go back to Herb and Jess. Herb is lost in his contrived world of not being sick. Emotionally, he is petrified of being sick. But publicly, he has not a care in the world. Internally, this relationship between the imagined and the real sets off biochemical chaos, upping his cortisol release and whatever emergency physiological and chemical responses are called for. Note also that Herb uses marijuana to regularly to "relax," so his biochemical picture is further complicated.

For Jess, the organizing factors are simply rage at her parents and fear. Beneath her promiscuous surface, her traumatic background is alive and persistent. She has been treated with ziprasidone followed by lamotrigine to manage her ever-present chaotic symptoms.

But, often in obscure ways, random experiences do reliably achieve organization. Constant bombardment of experiences, concrete and emotional, cohere. This exposition is not meant to assure you that we will always be able to come up with organizing principles for "#2" phenomena. It should, however, give you hope that we will be able to find our way within these situations.

Random Variables and How They Organize

32

Introduction

This chapter continues to address whether principles of organization can be discerned within random phenomena. Quantum mechanics and avant-garde jazz are examples. On inspection, organizing principles, no matter how obscure, can ultimately (and painstakingly) be discerned in these cases and probably all cases involving random phenomena.

Clinical events are difficult to predict. They are typically complicated in structure and subject to forces and events, the organization of which may be obscure (random in occurrence, not sequential). The trajectories of Jess' and Herb's treatments in the following chapter serve as illustrations.

The following is paraphrased (and shortened) from the engineering literature and reflects how random phenomena are treated there. It has been modified so it fits with this book and is as comprehensible as possible for non-engineers. As a function (a rule that gives value to a dependent variable that corresponds to specified values of one or more independent variables), a random variable is required to be measurable, allowing for probabilities to be assigned to sets of its potential values. It is common that the outcomes depend on some physical variables that are not predictable (or discernable). The domain of a random variable is a 'sample space,' which is interpreted as the set of possible outcomes of a random phenomenon. A random variable has a probability distribution. Random variables can be discrete, that is, take any of a specified finite or countable list of values characteristic of the random variable's probability distribution. This statement connects conceptually but loosely to the Heisenberg uncertainty principle, an axiom of quantum mechanics that may be simplified as there is a limitation to what one can know about the characteristics of a physical system, the position, momentum, and interaction of its atomic and subatomic particles including its constituent energy expressed in quanta.

Now that's truly a mouthful, but if you think about it, it makes sense. Random phenomena/variables in contrast to quanta of energy are measurable and plottable. If you want to plot them, you need to know the complicated rules governing their behavior (often quite obscure), and these are always there no matter how obscure. Note the analogy to avant-garde jazz. Initially, it may make no sense to the listener and has no apparent melody to tie it together. But just keep listening and you will begin to recognize a sophisticated musical structure.

Think of human experience and its lack of predictability. The troublesome factors, when not physical (measurable) are generally associated with emotions. Scientists often find it convenient to dismiss these presences as extraneous. After all they are not as rule bound and are only predictable within limits.

We will move now to clinical situations where randomness in the sequence of events is likely to be the rule when these events are viewed closely. Recognize that to make these situations comprehensible and ultimately manageable we frequently impose our own, often arbitrary, order onto them. This order is often idiosyncratic, reflective of the subject's convictions or mood. The result, as stated earlier in book when discussing heuristics, may be a personalization (falsification), of that clinical situation.

Further Reading:

The Randomness of Clinical Events (Stochastic Phenomena)

Blasband RA. The ordering of random events by emotional expression. Explore (NY). 2007;3(3):294.

Kriegel U. Subjective consciousness: a self-representational theory. London: Oxford University Press; 2011.

Marsh JK, Zeveney AS, De Los RA. Informant discrepancies in judgments about change during mental health treatments. Clin Psychol Sci. 2020;8(2):318–32.

Sage AP, Melsa JL. An introduction to probability and stochastic processes. Mineola: Dover Publications; 2013.

Smokler HE. Studies in subjective probability. 2nd ed. Melbourne: Krieger Publishing; 1980.

Clinical Judgment

33

Introduction

A good clinician, a master at using clinical data and well-constructed algorithms, should nonetheless not be overly bound by established doctrine. He or she presumably has plenty of clinical judgment in reserve. Clinical judgment is not just, or even primarily, based on doctrine, but instead on clinical and life experience.

Formal methods for accumulating and evaluating clinical data bear a resemblance to the way a good clinician works: accumulating and evaluating data, applying it, and being cognizant of and testing out results. But, even these methods have their deficiencies and may miss subtle, although influential, factors such as variations in the patient's personal circumstances and /or mood and the clinical impact of the treater's personality and preferences.

In Chapter 37, we will temporarily shift gears and touch on big data, machine language, and artificial intelligence, where data is compiled in large quantities. Computerized operations utilizing big data and artificial intelligence have their limitations but bear a resemblance to the way a good clinician accumulates and processes data.

Clinical Illustrations: Herb and Jess (2)

Clinical Illustrations: Herb and Jess

Herb and Jess are waiting in the wings, and we should return to them. Jess was sent to a "therapeutic" boarding school for 6 months. Herb attended seminars intended to instill a healthier attitude. Neither made a dent. The "#1" variable issues were clear in each case, for Herb pain and progressive disablement, and for Jess rebelliousness and promiscuity presumably at least partially the consequence of early and ongoing relationship disruptions and parental mishandling. In both cases, life was unmanageable. Conventional attempts at treatment, medical and psychiatric, were hardly successful.

Noncentral, "#2" variables were excluded from therapeutic explorations by their providers. For Herb, these included his need to please his wife and bolster his image for both his wife and himself. For Jess, these included her inexorable quest to find a boyfriend who could give her hope and essentially be her savior. Focusing on these issues might have been more successful in helping these patients to find order in their essentially chaotic experience [1, 2].

The central, organizing principle(s) may be concrete or intangible, but it is (they are) there. If we were to plot the "#1" variables in each case, we probably could come up with a statistical regression model that reflects the behavior of individual components or of all combined. And here is the point: as abstract as this exposition may sound, it is exactly what we as clinicians do all day in our offices. We semiautomatically consider all or most of the variables making up the current clinical situation. We assign clinical change that we believe is likely to occur, and we act accordingly. Over time, we reassess the situation to see how it is developing.

Herb almost died from disease progression and organ failure as it affected his kidneys and heart. Had he acknowledged his frailty sooner, the damage might have been mitigated. Jess was arrested for driving while under the influence of drugs and alcohol and refused to return to the psychotherapist from whom she appeared to be inseparable years earlier. The situations were chaotic based on external factors ("#2" variables). Fundamental, organizing clinical issues, Herb's terror of being ill and Jess' need to resist authority were clearly there. They provided organization for these chaotic cases even if they predisposed to their pathological outcomes.

References

1. Allan P. Coherence, chaos, and evolution in the social context. Futures. 1994;26(6):583–97.
2. Bruckner E, Ebeling E, Scharnhorst A. Stochastic dynamics of instabilities in evolutionary systems. Syst Dyn Rev. 1989;5(2):176–91.

Part XII

Clinical Judgment

[Part Introduction: Clinical judgment is the bedrock of the clinical process. Its successful application requires all of a clinician's learned and innate skills. Good clinical judgment requires excellent clinical training/skills but to a large extent its emergence is spontaneous, based both on experience and intuition. The product is steeped both in subjectivity (a well-developed feeling for the clinical process) and objectivity.]

Introduction

The issue addressed in this chapter involves the reliability of information recorded and processed by the clinician (in this case a psychotherapist), and clinical judgments based on this information. The clinical situation is subject to random (stochastic) events, emanating from both within and outside of the patient. As these events occur new clinical hypotheses are formulated. The clinician needs to proceed with humility, realizing that even with the benefit of statistical support, clinical decisions are never error-free.

Jess and Herb continue to serve as illustrations of randomness in patient and clinician's clinical choice. Discerning principles of organization within this seeming random collection of variables and their interactions is the focus of this chapter.

In an earlier chapter, we discussed cognitive processes, Kahneman's type 1 and type 2, involved in clinical decision-making. To retain clarity, we have relabeled these Kahneman type A and type B. We emphasized the importance of being aware of possible biases and reasoning errors as we work with clinical material. We also indicated that vignettes and patient examples like those used in this text (case-based learning) may represent the best ways to facilitate improved clinical decision-making despite their informality and innate imperfections (Kahneman type A).

The term "clinical judgment" is bandied about as if we all know what it means. There is a fat fly in my room just now. I can see it and follow it, but I cannot catch it. I've tried and tried. It has a "complicated" body, eyes, and multiple antennae. Intuitively, it seems like I should be able to predict its trajectory. But it keeps getting away from me. Can't be caught.

Clinical Illustration: Jess (2)

Prediction in Clinical Work

How could Jess' psychotherapist have predicted her impulsive flight after she had been so committed to the therapy? All indications were that she would stay unconditionally involved with him. When her father pressed her on her plans, she was quite clear. Her therapist was her "savior." She had worked with him for years, sometimes erratically but mostly unfailingly.

Uh-oh. Not so fast. There is more. Jess recently became convinced she had "psychic powers." These came under the heading of "empath." Empaths believe they can accurately sense emotions in others, pain and happiness included. As her new identity evolved, Jess progressively seemed to become truly empathetic, concerned about others and their welfare. And with this development, she paradoxically began to grow ever more independent.

At about the same time, she started missing therapy appointments and grew less interested in pleasing her parents and her therapist. Her therapist was impressed by her "growth," however. The change seemed real to him, and he believed it would progress and represented a kind of "conversion experience" for this previously self-centered 26-year-old. She also became involved with Aaron, a "perfectly wonderful human being." All rosy and according to her therapist reflecting a state of mind she had thoughtfully arrived at.

I hope you are feeling lost. I certainly am. We will let you know about the outcome in a moment. After all, what could be better. A previously "lost" young woman who was "transformed," a version of "Amazing Grace." At first, she was "lost" and now she was "found."

Oh yes, the conclusion. Well, it was not so pretty. Our "found" empath was soon arrested for "driving under the influence" (DUI). She had relinquished the main support in her life, her psychotherapist. She was back to zigging and zagging just like the fly. In contrast, the fly seemed to stick to its purpose, finding food and not getting swatted. Jess was unable to do anything like that on a consistent basis.

Randomness in Clinical Work

How random is Jess' behavior? Probably not fundamentally. Her actions just *appear* to be random in part because her motivations are multiple and intersect. The rest of the story is worth telling. A few months after she received her DUI, Jess' father had a stroke. The father and his wife (Jess' second adoptive mother) had moved to Montana and Jess (because of lack of money) moved with them. So, there was a new organizing principle in Jess' life: urgency. In this case, everyone was able to pull together around the father's medical condition, and Jess could at least temporarily give up her erratic behavior. Urgency and emergency are "#2" factors that are reliable in bringing behavior under control.

Governing principles (that are reliable like gravity or entropy) bring order to complicated behavior. This order may be partially illusory or at least fleeting. Of note, while the behavior of random (stochastic) variables calls for the discovery of organizing principles, identifying these principles may not lead to certainty. Attempts to find order in situations with large numbers of variables and prodigious amounts of data can be dealt with using computer technology, including artificial intelligence. This technology looks for and compares patterns. But, as will be discussed, these computer techniques have their limitations based on their lack of flexibility.

Return to "clinical judgment," an activity that organizes an assortment of clinical variables. You simply do not, like the psychoanalysts of old, want to claim that your clinical judgment is irrefutably accurate. In case this admonition seems unnecessary, think of how often patients receive inaccurate diagnoses based strictly on their clinician's experience and judgment. Jess encountered that kind of certainty on multiple occasions. It is painful to recall the mix of diagnoses that led to her being sent to two different residential treatment facilities, both with remarkably sophisticated leadership. During the first week at the first facility, the staff delivered a diagnostic opinion of "PTSD with occasional psychotic episodes." At the second, the "definitive" assessment had her as "sociopathic."

Getting It Right

So, what should we do to "get it right?" Here are some suggestions (Table 34.1):

This method of information exchange provides what we have come to call, clinical "truing." At each moment in a collaborative interaction, subtle data is exchanged and processed. This exchange may include information not likely to be revealed through a formal interview or questionnaire. In Jess' case, information about her idealized boyfriend Aaron can serve as an example:

- C (clinician): Jess tell me about Aaron.
- J (Jess): I love him. He is so wonderful.
- C: But the arguments you describe?
- J: They happen sometimes but he doesn't mean to hurt me.
- C: Tell me about his past relationships with women.
- J: His last girlfriend broke up with him because he was always drinking.
- C: What makes you say he is "wonderful," then?

Table 34.1 Getting It Right:

- Include nonspecific "#2" variables in your clinical formulation for the sake of incorporating nuance and for completeness.

    (a) For example, in Herb's case, there is his pride and fear of having a disease.

    (b) For Jess, there are the vestiges of past separations and traumas that have adulterated her relationships and made them untrustworthy and sometimes seem dangerous.

    (c) Finally, are the imperfections of the diagnoses themselves. Diagnoses are based on group data and may not closely fit the person to whom they are applied.

    (d) Added is that diagnoses may be applicable at first but lose accuracy over time.

- Access research literature.

- Collaborate with the patient and others in his or her life such as friends or family members.

The Remainders

We want to understand how often and in what ways "#2" variables and unsubstantiated narrative reporting enter into clinical judgment. The inclusion (and prevalence) of "#2" variables invariably muddy clinical judgment because of their imprecision. However, "#1" variables without consideration of "#2" variables do not sufficiently reflect the complexity of the clinical field and when used exclusively may misrepresent it. Sound clinical judgment requires both sources of clinical data, formal and personal. Herb's pride compromises him and distorts the course of his treatment. For Jess, a complicating factor may be her PTSD expressed as distrust of certain people and leading her to be untrustworthy in response. In each case, a clinical approach based on the recognition of both types of information, formal and impressionistic, is called for.

Here is an example of clinical reasoning based on both kinds of input. An assertion was made by her therapist that Jess was suffering from the "fear of disintegration of self" may be in ways correct. However, disintegration of self is a nonspecific category and limited in its utility. What then do we know to help explain Jess' chaotic life trajectory? Trustworthy relationships were not much in evidence through her adolescence. The stuff out of which her life was being built was shabby. Her first adoptive mother simply didn't like her. The second adoptive mother brought a "mirror, mirror on the wall who is the fairest of us all" attitude with her. OK, little "empathic attunement" + maternal rejection + narcissistic mother. But are you sure these are the actual building blocks of her scattered life? Shouldn't we include her well-meaning but devoted father in our formulation? All these explanations are based on clinical observation and logic. The point is that no matter how you cut it, whether your clinical impression and judgment are based on established facts (concrete findings) or psychologically justified formulations, there is plenty of room for error.

Restatement

Jess is shaky. She had inadequate parenting. Her parents couldn't really understand her needs and insisted on compliance while not being able to earn it from her through their comprehension of her needs. We can be relatively certain of this formulation in part because Jess would agree with it. The formulation also is consistent with other clinical developments including Jess' overuse of alcohol after the loss of her boyfriend. Once her drinking and romance with, yes, cocaine, was uncovered, she became increasingly "lost."

Our Opinion Given the Data

Jess indeed needed a solid relationship to sustain her. In part, or perhaps largely, this requirement was based on parenting deficiencies. She had been "re-parented" by her psychotherapist who could comfortably say he regarded Jess like a daughter. The basis of this statement is the observations made by her psychotherapist and is rooted in several years of interpersonal attention through psychotherapy. During most of these years, our zigzagging fly (Jess) mostly moved in a predictable trajectory. Toward the end, it lost its way.

Later in the book, we will again talk about other means for making sense of data generated from complex clinical situations. For example, computerized methods such as artificial intelligence typically yield a multitude of data. For now, it may be helpful to reiterate that computers are largely restricted to concrete manipulation of data. Making inferences is not reliably their domain. Clinical work is not neat, precise, or static. To get reliable results, one needs to maintain this perspective and realize that it is helpful to see random clinical situations as having "minds of their own." You, the clinician, are not the master of the clinical situation, even in the seemingly most clear-cut medical-social situation. Making predictions using available data is a good thing. Believing that you can accurately predict is often self-deceptive.

Clinical Judgment, Illustrated

35

Introduction

In this chapter, brief examples from prior case histories are presented to illustrate the formulation and application of clinical judgment. Especially when dealing with imprecise "#2" variables, there are limited "cookbook" formulas for making precise clinical decisions. Nevertheless, there are usually principles that can guide clinicians as they make these decisions. Clinical algorithms are often designed to provide such guidance although, of necessity, they address clinical categories rather than specific cases.

So, how does a clinician know what to do next with all this "zigging and zagging", "#2" variables now prominently included in the mix? He or she starts with a "case" that is described by demographics, symptoms, and history. These "#1" variables are familiar and invite the use of clinical algorithms. For diabetes mellitus and most other clinical conditions, prescribed diagnostic procedures include a clinical examination, history, review of (organ) systems, laboratory studies, and diagnostic imaging. Putting it all together and moving beyond the apparent clarity of "#1" variables and the most basic algorithmic derived plan, the clinical process may not be as straightforward as hoped for. Later, once clinical judgment is introduced, certainty yields, at least partially, to guesswork.

Clinical Illustrations: SAF and Others

Here's an example. I (SAF) have been having "balance issues." I am in my 70s and as distressing as it was to acknowledge I had to concede that my age was probably "catching up" to me. So, I did what was logical and consulted with a neurologist.

Clinical Examples: SAF and Others

S. A. Frankel et al., *Complexity in Health Care*,
https://doi.org/10.1007/978-3-031-14949-8_35

Following an MRI, nerve conduction study, and meeting with a physical medicine specialist, there were no concrete findings (despite one additional fall during this process due to loss of balance). I was also referred to a physical therapist, Alan, who I thought was unimpressive and spoke broken English. I want to emphasize that my physicians were all well-respected and willing to spend extra time on my problem. From there, I was referred to a foot and ankle specialist whose contribution was to notice that my calf muscles were "tight."

Of course, you've figured out by now that it was Alan who ultimately saved the day. The neurologist discussed surgery and onabotulinumtoxin A (abbreviated "Botox") for assisting with muscle loosening, but Alan offhandedly rejected both choices because of potential complications. Instead, he put his experience and judgment to work and prescribed a few "dumb" but challenging stretching exercises. Honestly, they were so simple that it was almost embarrassing. But I was in trouble and needed help, so I committed myself to following his recommendations.

The outcome? I'm not back to dancing (in my youth, I won a few dance contests) but I am ever so slowly regaining my flexibility and balance. At each point, with me resisting, the physical therapist called the shots, and he invariably has been right. How did he know what to do next? I wish I knew. He does understand muscles and their anatomy and functioning. Clearly, that background was necessary for him to choose exercises and instruct me to use them. But there is more and that is what I'm calling "clinical judgment."

Clinical judgment that incorporates clinical experience but goes beyond it is a key "#2" variable. It is hard to quantify, but often recognizable. Notice how we are breaking down the clinical situation into its component but as in this case often hard to define parts.

Herb's physician's judgment was that his support for Herb's desire to hide his diagnosis from his wife was required to retain Herb's commitment to treatment. Eventually, he believed that Herb was ready to hear the full truth about his illness and Herb was able to tell his wife about it. Jess' psychotherapist prior to Jess' slide into alcohol dependence relied heavily on clinical judgment from his years-long treatment relationship with her. He was incessantly challenged by her adoptive mother whose underlying motive seemed to be to prove that Jess was damaged and not worth spending the money on for her repair. His judgment was based on his view that the disrupted parenting bond explained much of Jess' deviant behavior. Once the family moved from California to Montana, and the father had his stroke, his hold on Jess started to slip.

The point about clinical judgment, as illustrated by both these situations, is that there are no algorithms for definitive guidance. Why does one clinician, like Alan, get it right, while others with the same information and similar clinical tools have poor results?

Connecting the dots: (1) much activity in a clinical situation is at least partially random (the fly!); (2) within this apparent randomness, there likely are unifying principles that may, however, remain obscure; (3) part of the elusiveness of this situation is explained by the fact that "#2" variables populate this, and in fact all, clinical situations and are imprecise; and (4) apart from gleaning the opinions of experienced clinicians who can attempt to rate the clinical importance (weight) of each variable, there may be no readily applicable way to quantify the contribution of each. Note that the term "factor" as used in "factor analysis" refers to a collection of variables that are correlated one with the other. There a "factor" (of which there is likely to be many) is one entity containing a collection of correlated individual variables.

Further Reading:

Critical Thinking and Clinical Judgment

Alfaro-LeFevre R. Critical thinking and clinical judgment: a practical approach to outcome - focused thinking. 4th ed. Philadelphia: Saunders; 2008.

Biklen D. The myth of clinical judgment. J Soc Issues. 1988;44(1):127–40.

Gambrill E. Critical thinking in clinical practice: improving the quality of judgments and decisions. 3rd ed. New York: Wiley; 2012.

Jackson M, Ignatavicius DD, Case B. Critical thinking and clinical judgment. New York: Springer; 2004.

Schalock RL. Outcome-based evaluation. 2nd ed. Dordrecht: Kluwer Academic/Plenum; 2001.

Schalock RL, Luckasson R. Clinical judgment. Washington, DC: American Association on Intellectual & Developmental Disabilities; 2005.

Cultural Values, i.e., Mores, Ethics, Standards, and Habits

36

Introduction

This chapter presents new subsets of "#2" variables, "#2a" and "#2b." Included in this category are variables associated with culture and values. The case of Kamile is rich in these values-laden components, including ingrained, culturally engendered habits.

As we near the end of our search for manifest-clearly defined ("#1") variables and ambiguous-hard to "pin down" ("#2") variables, we have also identified other groups of variables ("#3" variables and their subcategories) that earn their place because they are difficult to classify, i.e., may be microscopic or otherwise hard to define (may lack concrete form).

Start with those variables ("#2a") that are habitual, inculcated through repetition? They are "under your skin." You regard them as part of your being. While you might be aware of them in yourself, you aren't likely to reflect on them. They go by names like culture, beliefs including religious, "truths," customs, and just plain habits. These variables while amorphous are potentially quantifiable and can be subjected to operational definitions.

Habits and Mores

Regarding habits, today I (SAF) awoke at 7:30 A.M. In sequence, I went through a routine of drinking two glasses of cold water, showering, doing stretching exercises, extensive dental hygiene (while I boned up on statistics), greeting my dog Sherpa, eating a bowl of oatmeal, and drinking a full glass of soy milk. I'm very glad no one could observe me since I would feel silly about their viewing my routine. I am also glad that everything was in its proper place since if it hadn't been, I might have

---

Clinical Illustration: Kamile

spent excessive time to correct that. I always walk-jog for 30 minutes. I love spending time with my wife but there was only 10 minutes for that this morning. Holy mackerel, am I really telling you all this?

Certainly, habit and temperament are two influences that cannot be neglected. The impact of culture (and/or religion) contributing content for habit is often an afterthought for clinicians. Omar, from Saudi Arabia, who you met earlier, unendingly bargained with me. First, was my fee. He always paid me late or did what he could to avoid paying, never acknowledging he was planning to do that. He was not only looking for a bargain but was also alert to the possibility that I might cheat him. Yet, he seemed so honest and appreciative for my help. Fortunately, I had spent time in the Middle East and was aware that this behavior was not necessarily hostile, likely instead to be culturally based. The religious issue was there too. Omar, Muslim, and me, Jewish.

Culture, as a source for habit, includes more than religion. During my early years in the Bronx, we carried knives to "protect" ourselves. Fighting was part of the culture (although we did our best to avoid it). It was "Bronx culture," just as was perilously jumping on the back of a moving bus to get a free ride.

Keeping track of this subcategory of variables (including habit, culture, and religion) as they influence behavior is, of course, close to impossible. As discussed in the previous chapter, one statistical method for organizing variables associated with this this experience is through "factor analysis," lumping closely correlated variables into categories (factors). Clinically relevant factors of current interest to us might include motivation, background, intellectual ability, and mood including enthusiasm and discouragement.

Subsets of "#2" Variables: "#2a" and "#2b"

For the sake of clarity, we have created two additional groups of "#2" variables. More subcategories will likely be created as we move along. To repeat the subcategories of "#2" variables are the following:

- "#2a", are habits of thought and behavior that may be culturally based, e.g., Omar.
- "#2b", variables are often related to motivation and emotion, e.g., Martin.

"#2a" and "#2b" variables are typically perceived as integrated with the fabric of the case, features that are hard to distinguish from presenting signs and symptoms.

"#3" Variables

We will further define "#3" variables and their subsets in the next section of this book. These will include (1) "entities" that are the product of the mind and (2) the microscopic/molecular building blocks of matter.

Kamile

All the represented "#2a" traits were relevant for Kamile at age 30. Kamile's father, who died when she was 10, had been well-known for his theatrical achievements and his successes significantly burdened Kamile. In contrast, she perceived herself as a "loser." For the most part, Kamile was humorless. Trustworthy to the hilt. At age 25, she was still eager each summer to travel with her admirable but lackluster family. They regularly went to a cabin in northern British Columbia. She was smart (as corroborated by neuropsychological testing). But she had no ambition other than to excel at the adventure game, Dungeons and Dragons (D&D). She was a creative "dungeon master" who lived and breathed D&D. As a challenging adventure game, D&D has high status within a segment of the adolescent-young adult community.

Kamile was difficult to work with. She was judgmental. She rejected pleasure. She resisted personal warmth and acceptance. We can give her a diagnosis. High-functioning autism (currently a part of the autism spectrum disorder, DSM-5 299.00) comes to mind; at another time in DSM history, she might have been called "schizoid." In this case, it may be best at the start at the end of the story. Kamile after several years of psychiatric treatment, at first with medication and then emphasizing psychotherapy, has emerged as neither Asperger's syndrome nor as having a schizoid personality disorder. Instead, she has inexplicably "grown up."

Kamile's metamorphosis, like Nafi's, was surprising and at least in part mysterious. This is the way it is with "#2" variables. It is often difficult to tell what exactly has worked but not hard to know that something positive has happened. The following statement is paraphrased from Kamile's psychiatrist. Kamile was "suffering". Her contemptuousness was apparently a "thin cover" for despair. In effect, she had given up. Why try when life is "so miserable?" Like many smart adolescents, she was hyperaware of her mortality and the "senselessness" of chronic suffering deriving from life's travails. Dungeons and Dragons scenarios were more than just imaginative forays. They were an escape into a fantasy world that seemed almost entirely real to Kamile. By not challenging this choice, her parents were complicit.

"Deep down" Kamile imagined that her future existence would be no different from that of her mother's and stepfather's. She was destined to drift into obscurity, "go nowhere." No one could help her modify her outlook since all family members had the same hopeless perspective. Kamile's world was bleak, Kamile was bleak, Dungeons and Dragons offered great adventures, but in the end, it was only a game.

The problem was that there seemed to be no escape. Kamile's routine was compelling; going beyond it was frightening for her. Being curious about anyone else's life was out. Everything in Kamile's life was colored by her lack of imagination and seeming stubbornness. You certainly would not want to be trapped on a desert island with Kamile.

To understand how Kamile moved beyond her lack of flexibility and dominating imagination, it is important to recall that "#2" variables work in sync with other variables. Other influences, e.g., "#2a" and "#2b" variables or the later described

"#3" variables, are likely to be there but often hidden. And there may be other yet unidentified clinically relevant factors at work. This idea may be the clue to why stubborn, hard-to-change personality traits can at times be made to yield. After several costly missteps due to "foot dragging," Kamile was admitted to a California university. To attend she had to commute to San Francisco daily. The commute was challenging, as was finding her way around the school and its requirements. Like it or not, Kamile was forced to be with people she had previously rejected. Honestly, she had to admit they were not so bad, and to her horror, she found herself enjoying many of them. These were the "superficial" people who she had always avoided.

But, why now? What made it possible for her to override her schizoid tendencies and suddenly come alive? I've been watching my 3-year-old grandson Nathan and 2-year-old granddaughter Ayla repeat each new act multiple times. Of course, Piaget defined this developmentally relevant behavior as involving "circular reactions," part of what it takes to master a task. It is interesting to see what happens to these actions as they become incorporated into Nathan's broader repertoire. In part, they are joined to more complex patterns, but they also remain, the parts still observable in the resulting synthetic behaviors.

Kamile apparently never unlearned the habits she formed early. Here is the tricky part. Some people are reasonably quick to unlearn habits and others are not. It would be reasonable to think of this inequity in addiction terms. It seems that some people are biologically wired to be addictive, mindlessly following established patterns of behavior and others less so. Maybe this is part of what we mean by temperament, the biological part of habit.

But then, why did Kamile begin to shed her "shell" when she started studying at university? There are two tentative explanations. Number one, this was the first time she encountered anything about which she could feel passionate. In her case, it was the new prospect of preparing for a career in film, creating special effects. There is no etiological explanation for why this subject would evoke such passion. But it did. Number two, for the first time in her life, she was on her own, exposed to a world outside of her home and family.

These habit-breaking experiences match those Nafi encountered in his Mandarin Chinese class. Both Nafi and Kamile had been "sheltered" as children and were adored by their parents. In both cases, there was little to attract them away from the comfort of parents and habits. There is a strong identity between associated variables in both cases: parents, home, comfort, and habits. Both Kamile and Nafi encountered a habit-breaking experience that stood in sharp contrast to other cherished habitual ways of being.

"#3" Variables: Introduction

"#3" variables contribute to the potpourri of remaining clinical variables. The concept "variable" may be unclear when cloaked in mathematical-statistical language. For the sake of clarity, definitions of a "variable" include its being a "factor, trait, or condition" that is likely to change and can exist in different amounts or types within a single task. A common feature of these definitions is variability and "change."

Typically, when included in scientific determinations, variables are separated into those that are considered "independent, dependent, or controlled." In each case, the magnitude of the variable in part depends on its relationship to the other variables making up that part of the clinical field.

In mathematics, a variable is a quantity that can assume any value from a set of values. When unspecified, it may be characterized as "unknown" or "indeterminate." When specified, it may take the form of a "parameter" (a quantity that is part of the input for a problem and remains constant when used in the solution to the problem), coefficient, or a constant, or it may be a random variable associated with statistical probability (Oxford English Dictionary, Oxford Press, 2006).

Part XIII

"#3" Variables

[Part Introduction: At the completion of this part of the book, we will have concluded our inventory of the content and structure of complex clinical situations. One apology. There turn out to be too many categories for comfort. We did not start expecting this. But just think. Several of our categories are concerned with ambiguous variables ("#2" variables), exist solely in the mind of the patient, and/or are too small to be seen by the naked eye. These all need to be included since, because as stated earlier in the book, otherwise your description of a patient and his or her experience will be anemic. If you remove any one of these categories your construction will not be true to life. Can you really remove the microscopic/molecular level or epigenetic contributions and adequately understand the patient's presentation and treatment needs? In this part, we discuss these more esoteric contributions to the clinical picture, including those from epigenetics.]

A New Category, "#3" Variables, Beyond the Elusiveness of "#2" Variables

37

Introduction

In this chapter, we further develop the concepts of "#3" variables. "#3" variables have two subclassifications: "#3a" and "#3b". "#3a" variables are microscopic and cannot be seen by the naked eye such as genes, genetic-related propensities, and associated molecular structure. "#3b" variables consist of beliefs and mental constructions that exist in the minds of the patient and/or clinician often without counterparts in the physical world. In this chapter, as in clinical situations, these variable sets are combined with "#1" and "#2" variables to describe a patient, Londyn. To be accurate, a clinician's clinical reasoning must be augmented by recognition of these subtle, generally hard to detect but potentially influential "#3" variables.

Now to go further into the "never-never land" of variables and their effect on clinical outcome. For this chapter, we need to consider variables that are thus far excluded from our model. It would be strange if our original two-category ("#1" and "#2" variables) model included all possible categories of variables. To expand this list, we need to go back to the clinical situation as it is, immersing ourselves as if we are deep-sea diving and looking at a multitude of unfamiliar objects.

Added variable subcategories:
"#3a" variables are building blocks of clinical reality that like the microscopic features of behavior may include the following:
1. The biochemistry and neurotransmission that govern our biology and for the most part cannot be observed by the naked eye.
2. Genetic propensities influencing behavior such as an individual's response to stress and his or her innate social traits. These capabilities are regulated by the epigenome, i.e., the genetic "control center" for humans.

Clinical Illustration: Londyn

© The Author(s), under exclusive license to Springer Nature Switzerland AG 2023
S. A. Frankel et al., *Complexity in Health Care*,
https://doi.org/10.1007/978-3-031-14949-8_37

"#3b" variables are those poorly defined entities of belief and thought that like habits simply exist in the mind of the subject or are shared between people.

Each of these categories/subcategories is legitimately a clinical variable.

Londyn

Take Londyn, a seemingly well-adjusted, college educated 35-year-old. In her early 20s, she was delightful, smart, humorous, and forgiving. At age 25, she moved from San Francisco to Seattle, excited about "starting" her adult life. But despite the excellence of the "raw material," it wasn't long before she was floundering. At first, at age 30, she thought she wanted to become an electrical engineer but for unexplained reasons abruptly dropped that goal. She had been popular as a friend with the boys in college but did not continue relationships with any of them. The remaining ones were "losers" according to her. So far, none of these developments, taking place over about 5 years, followed an expectable developmental trajectory. By then, at age 35, she was dragging herself through graduate school having reluctantly chosen to become a mid-level technician, a profession that clearly was beneath her original aspirational goal.

What is the point of making these distinctions? More angels on the head of a pin, or what? Here is the answer. Lumping all these "definers" together completes the "real" nature of the clinical situation, filling in how it is constructed.

Londyn did not thrive. By age 35, she was looking haggard, her sparkling sense of humor was gone, and she had forsworn competing for virtually anything. There was no systemic illness ("#1" variable) and ostensibly no complicating life events. Stuck and sad, Londyn finally went to a psychotherapist who claimed to have spiritual capabilities. After 2 years of this treatment, Londyn was no better. Now she was 37 years old and not far from being biologically "up against the clock." She was not just beginning to lose her sparkle but in effect had become a chronic patient, now making the rounds of physical medicine, acupuncturists, and spiritual healing all to deal with her loss of motivation and newly acquired back pain. She had moved from being a marvel to a mess.

At age 37, many treatments tried; none helpful. At this point, Londyn, who had been against psychotropic medication, gave in. She discovered that her health plan would support visits to a psychiatrist. With all other options exhausted, she yielded. She would try psychotropic medication. Her previous psychotherapist who was biased against psychotropic medication warned against this choice. But Londyn was desperate. Having graduated from school, she took an uninspiring job as a mid-level technician. The rules and regulations governing her work were maddening and she "dreaded" work from day to day.

There were physical problems as well. She developed chronic back pain and learned that she had a BRAC2 gene mutation, predisposing her to breast cancer. Now there was more to be concerned about (note that the genetic mutation BRAC1 has a poorer prognosis than the analogous mutation, BRAC2)—loss of motivation, social withdrawal, chronic back pain, and risk of breast cancer. But, apart from chronic pain and the BRAC2 gene mutation, there actually were no "#1" issues. Her life had progressed quite well in her mid-20s. Spiritual guidance was "nice" but not helpful. Psychotherapy was the same.

The psychiatrist she saw seized on the idea that she was clinically depressed (diagnosis assigned was Major Depressive Disorder DSM-5 296.20-36). He prescribed venlafaxine ER beginning at 75 mg/day, slowly building to 225 mg/day. For about 4 months, she felt less depressed and more energized. However, this state of mind was short-lived, and she required several dose increases. Venlafaxine is associated with a severe withdrawal syndrome that can include "brain zaps," headaches, nausea, nightmares, and irritability. Later, when withdrawal was attempted, Londyn experienced all these symptoms making the withdrawal process protracted and difficult. Eventually, venlafaxine was discontinued and a more tolerable regimen with another antidepressant, bupropion, was established.

Missing variables. A "#1" variable in this case likely included a personality trait, Londyn's tendency to underestimate herself. "#2" variables may have included the effect of aging and the impact of learning about her genetic mutation. But these factors were neither confirmed as specific provocations nor linked to distinct symptoms. "#3" variables could now be hypothesized to help explain Londyn's profound collapse. It wouldn't be far-fetched to imagine as etiological an undiagnosed neurological syndrome. Many factors including medication and nutrition can affect biological outcome by influencing one's epigenome to activate or inactivate genes affecting mood or behavior. However, we do not have enough information about Londyn at this point to implicate a genetic basis for her symptoms.

Temperament. Back to Londyn. Originally, she simply appeared depressed. It would have been neat if that had been the whole picture. However, that didn't seem to be the case. A biological given shaping her personality was temperament. Temperament is hard to define except through its effect. Londyn reacted sharply to most experiences. When happy she was "on top of the world" but when disappointed her mood dropped sharply. These episodes were not like hypomanic/manic and major depressive episodes of bipolar disorder since they did not occur cyclically. In part, it was simply the way she was. Looking at her situation retrospectively, one could infer that something out of the ordinary was happening to this reactive young woman, putting her in a repeatedly negative mood.

An Unexpected Influence

A possible answer and a reasonable candidate to explain her evolving difficulties is a new event in Londyn's life, introduced belatedly. Londyn's parents had divorced while she was in middle school and her mother went into an unremitting angry mood. Everything in her mother's life had turned from neutral to bad, Londyn included. Her mother and Londyn had been inseparable previously and now, according to the mother, "everything had turned to shit." Here complexity is increased by the timing of the introduction of a new variable. The divorce and Londyn's reaction to it takes us back to a not-so-subtle feature of this case, the introduction of a new "#1" (exogenous) variable, an event that had a profound impact on Londyn's mood and adjustment.

Clinical assessments. Real-life situations like this one are almost always more complex than they seem at first. New influences, including those that are biological and personal/interpersonal ("#3" variables), can be introduced at any point. Determinative events can include biochemical shifts and epigenetic influences. Biological (medical) testing and psychological/neuropsychological assessment may be used to help sort out and quantify the components.

Clinical Judgment, Revisited

To conclude this chapter, we return to the topic of clinical judgment. It has probably occurred to you that while it would be ideal to have definitive instructions for guiding clinical judgment, they simply do not exist. Regarding other means of arriving at certainty through formal assessment, we are part way there. For example, looking at the depth and precision of a complex ("projective") personality assessment like the Rorschach and R-PAS psychometric tests (which are less subjective than you might think) and the remarkable amount of detail available from radiological scans like an MRI, we have a lot of technology on our side. But the precision of psychological and neuropsychological assessments has limits, and the results from these assessments *do not* necessarily remain fully reflective of the patient's psychological functioning over time (e.g., findings from the Rorschach/R-PAS is in part dependent on the timing of administration), and diagnostic imaging, e.g., MRI, certainly can miss lesions and in part its interpretation depends on the skill of the radiologist who reads it.

Affective variables ("#2" variables) coloring a clinical situation may have multiple and at times pervasive clinical impacts potentially confounding any formal assessment. The clinician in his or her office is subject to an onslaught of clinical factors that includes "#1", "#2a", "#2b", "#2…", and "#3a", "#3b" variables, all directly impacting the patient and interacting with one another. Ideally, artificial intelligence (AI) might help organize complex clinical presentations like this. It has been shown repeatedly that computer-based programs like artificial intelligence in its present incarnation cannot replace clinician judgment, in part because artificial intelligence is limited in its ability to make inferences about clinical situations. AI is also limited in its ability to incorporate dimensionality, e.g., the place of motivation, in a clinical situation.

Table 37.1 List of the variables we have grouped

– "#1" variables that can be named, i.e., given an operational definition. Tend to be observable and defined

– "#2" variables lack clear and stable definitions. Manifestations may be multiple and fleeting. They are denotatively inexact

   – "#2a" variables refer to habitual behavior and may have a cultural theme

   – "#2b" variables refer to emotion, including motivation

– "#3" variables include those that constitute the building blocks of matter and experience

   – "#3a" variables are biological features of clinical reality including (i) features that are microscopic and (ii) genetic propensities influencing behavior. These variables are all associated with the epigenome

   – "#3b" variables are poorly defined aspects of belief and thought. These exist in the mind, are not concrete

When we began this analysis of the clinical field, collections of variables often seemed inherently amorphous, messy, and only partially separable into related groups. We have done our best to organize these. Here is a summary (Table 37.1):

Warning! Oversimplification is falsification. Simplifying a clinical picture is often necessary for practical reasons, e.g., in the form of heuristics such as assigning a diagnosis. However, simplification is likely to fail up close with the patient not recognizing him or herself through the assigned label(s).

Further Reading

List A: "#3" Variables—Existing in the Mind (Sociology)

Goffman E. The presentation of self in everyday life the presentation of self in everyday life. London, England: Penguin Classics; 2022.

Mead GH. Mind, self and society: from the standpoint of a social behaviorist. Chicago: University of Chicago Press; 1934.

List B: "#3" Variables—Microscopic Phenomena and the Products of One's Mind

Damasio A, Damasio H. How life regulation and feelings motivate the cultural mind: a neurobiological account. In: The Cambridge handbook of cognitive development. Cambridge: Cambridge University Press; 2022. p. 15–26.

Mukundan CR. Understanding and dealing with the mental creations: living in real and virtual worlds. J Psychol Clin Psychiatry. 2018;9(4):394–8.

Roy DP. Basic constituents of the visible and invisible matter - a microscopic view of the universe [Internet]. arXiv [physics.pop-ph]. 2000. http://arxiv.org/abs/physics/0007025.

Toward a Comprehensive Discussion of "#3" Variables

38

Introduction

The final addition to our list of variables, "#3" variables, includes those that constitute the building blocks of matter and experience. To be useful, this category will need to be precisely subclassified. The spectrum of manifestations is likely to be broad.

The "#3" variables remaining are in part the truly unseen ones including those making contributions to the genetic, epigenetic, biochemical, and associated neurological bases of clinical work. Many of these influences exist at the molecular level. As suggested, these are chemical in nature and include genetic and other biological processes impacting health.

Back to the consulting room. Thoughtful clinical judgment means going beyond "#1" variables. In working directly with the patient or in reviewing ancillary data, the clinician becomes aware of and cognizes elusive variables ("#2" variables and "#3" variables) that may be important but are easily missed. In so doing, she or he attends to subtle information from the patient including information conveyed nonverbally.

Kamile, continued

Return here to Kamile and her temperament. Why had she been so unimaginative, and habit bound? Her two years younger brother, who had been exposed to a similar home environment (nothing of note had happened in the family during Kamile's early life), was clearly less rigid than Kamile. So, what made it possible for her to change so rapidly over the course of only a year after entering college? Was the

---

Clinical Illustration: Kamile (2)

S. A. Frankel et al., *Complexity in Health Care*,
https://doi.org/10.1007/978-3-031-14949-8_38

potential for Kamile's developmental change simply biologically programmed or was it latent, ready to be unlocked through exposure to others as she grew older?

In keeping with the theme of this book, the answer may lie with a combination of factors. Note that in our opinion, the only way we can catalogue these influential factors is to unpack them through deconstruction. We have the following shortened list of items potentially influencing Kamile's development to choose from: (1) parenting; (2) unrecognized traumatic experiences (experience traumatic to one person is not necessarily traumatic to another); (3) temperament, e.g., emotional reactivity and predisposition for promiscuous bonding to others; (4) experiences that are obscure and not appreciated by others as impactful; (5) biological events, the importance of which are not yet recognized; (6) personal events like menarche that are biologically programmed and may be experienced as stressful; and (7) epigenetic factors influencing changes in the genome that regulate behavior.

There is an additional, so far excluded, factor and that may have been influential and essential for understanding Kamile. Like other girls, Kamile went through a sequence of hormonal and other biologically programmed steps as she matured. Not stated so far is that she didn't much like being a girl. She had heard a lot from parents about the risk of being sexualized by boys. Privately, these warnings frightened her. It got worse during puberty, starting with menarche. She did not like the idea that her breasts were enlarging. In her mind, she would become progressively vulnerable, especially as these body changes began to show. But this subject was taboo for Kamile. She could mouth the words but could not stand the thoughts. You can infer the rest.

Beginning in the fifth grade, Kamile began to isolate. She vowed to herself that she would not share her secret thoughts with anyone. Her emotional life became strained. But, to her unsuspecting (and emotionally restricted) parents, her withdrawal, while concerning, was mysterious.

How do "#1", "#2", and "#3" variables fit here, especially "#3" variables? It is simple. They come together as a tapestry. The threads are the "#3" variables. The most microscopic, but in ways the most fundamentally influential, components since their biological structure may have widespread relevance for health and adjustment altogether. "#2" variables provide movement and "color," while "#1" variables set the familiar themes for the case. What is so interesting is that no one of these three factors exist separately from the others. As an adult, Kamile made a tenuous but acceptable social adjustment, and Kamile's biology almost certainly includes a genetic predisposition classifying her for the autism spectrum (restrained affect, social isolation, and her obsession with Dungeons and Dragons, a complicated adventure game involving multiple players and a leader, the "dungeon master"). It would be reasonable to think of her progression as involving a personal system repeatedly striving for expression with affect moving toward the center as she learns to appreciate its significance.

Sorry, of course you can see through our simplifications. But the model is practical. For our current purpose, we do well to note that biological influence, in part genetic and epigenetic in origin, likely colors the entire picture.

Part XIV

The Empirical-Collaborative (E-C) Method

[Part Introduction: You probably have been asking how we intend to substantiate our understanding of clinical situations. How do we know we are on the right track? Our choice is to use and extend standard logic-based operations, namely, induction, deduction, and add a new category, "abduction" for this purpose. In this way we not only can substantiate our understanding but also expand on it. Our method is illustrated in the next several chapters under the heading "empirical-collaborative (E-C) method."]

39

The Empirical-Collaborative Method, Our Method for Using Clinical Data to Arrive at a Paradigm Shift for Clinical Practice

Introduction

This chapter begins to elaborate our "empirical-collaborative (E-C)" method. We do that in the case of Erin by illustrating its use for unpacking a long-held family secret, and for Kamile through its use in clarifying her diagnosis. The use of this method is detailed in subsequent chapters. The E-C method uses deductive and inductive reasoning, as well as a less well-known logical technique known as abduction (involving extrapolation) for discovery of obscure or hidden data in a clinical situation.

The Empirical-Collaborative Method, Further Explored

We hope you can discern the method to our madness as we describe our clinical process for ferreting out subtle, often unacknowledged, factors involved in clinical work. We have been relying on case examples to illustrate our work. How to use them for analyzing complex clinical situations? What do Juliana, Seth, Omar, our diabetic patients, the schizophrenic woman from Yemen, Herb (polyarteritis nodosa), Boris, Nafi, Maggie, Ben, Londyn, Jess, Erin, Martin, and Kamile have in common? None of these cases are much out of the ordinary for physicians. Some are medically complicated, while others not. All are complex, however, when the "#1", "#2", "#2a", "#2b", "#3a", and "#3b" variables in each case are considered.

What will it take for us to get to the point where our response to unpacking a confounding clinical situation is not to throw our hands up and again simplify through familiar diagnostic and algorithmic shortcuts? In contrast, we want to devise a method for deconstructing each case and arranging the pieces in some kind of order that allows for reasonably precise treatment planning and execution. Also, we want to substantiate our interest in clinical complexity and make the case that without this perspective (a full appreciation for the complexity of each case), one is likely to miss important diagnostic and prognostic clues.

S. A. Frankel et al., *Complexity in Health Care*,
https://doi.org/10.1007/978-3-031-14949-8_39

We call this method "empirical-collaborative" since it prompts us to use our clinical data to review the case and deconstruct it.

- For example, Kamile's case seems straightforward. Autistic spectrum disorder or schizoid personality disorder. She comes from a conventional family, all members perhaps affectively blunted. No factors that could be considered traumatic are obvious. Add the possible contribution of Kamile's continual confrontation with the "real world" after an upbringing marked by unrelenting parental pampering and the clinical picture begins to fill in.
- We return to a previously discussed case, Erin. Exploration with Erin and her parents surprisingly revealed that Erin had been born without a uterus and was missing a kidney. Neither she nor her parents initially discussed this information with Erin's psychotherapist, and her primary care physician did not weigh in during the initial psychiatric workup. Apparently, her parents minimized this topic because it was so distressing to them.

The issue now is devising a method for unpacking clinical data, especially the "silent" data tucked into a dense array of clinical information. With Kamile, for example, we started with a presumptive diagnosis of "high-functioning" autism or schizoid personality disorder. Schizoid personality disorder ultimately seemed more descriptive of Kamile's temperament and behavior, so we've chosen to focus on the ICD-10 definition of schizoid personality disorder. Summarized from ICD-10 schizoid personality disorder includes the following (the analogous DSM 5 category is 301.20):

- Choosing few activities that provide pleasure
- Limited capacity to express emotions
- Apparent indifference to praise or criticism
- Little interest in sexual experiences
- Prefers to be alone
- Preoccupation with fantasy life
- Lack of close friends
- Uninterested in prevailing social norms

Fits well for a start. We could leave it at that, except that Kamile was atypical in other ways. From the beginning, in contrast to her bland affect, she seemed to devour psychotherapy, clamoring for more time with her psychotherapist. She quickly becomes attached to him and her primary care physician as well.

In addition, there was "soft" information about her development that did not fit the schizoid category. Her social discomfort appears to have developed in the context of a devoted albeit socially (as opposed to personally) isolated family. The family was not lacking in intimacy. Her parents doted on Kamile. However, the outside world was experienced as hostile and at times dangerous by family members, an attitude presumably restricting Kamile's motivation to expand socially. But her home was not devoid of warmth.

And there are other incongruities. What to make of Kamile's insistent disinterest in sex and repudiation of her gender? As she moved through adolescence, she became strident about this subject. Also, while disinterest in school complemented her social avoidance, it did not match her remarkable aptitude which had been confirmed by neurocognitive testing.

The Empirical-Collaborative Method Illustrated

40

Introduction

This chapter illustrates the use of the empirical-collaborative method with a patient, Ben, to demonstrate the unpacking of the clinical information the patient was having difficulty revealing.

Ben

Here we take a close look at Ben, noting the plethora of variables that make up his material (formal) and personal clinical situation. These variables are listed in (Table 40.1):

Notice the abundance of variables, many dissimilar, constituting Ben's formal and personal situation. Key steps in the empirical-collaborative approach are delineated.

Table 40.1 Variables associated with Ben's clinical situation

- Symptoms supporting a "major depressive disorder" (ICD-10, F32) diagnosis
- Supplementary descriptive variables, e.g., smart, handsome, cultured, restricted in emotional expressiveness
- As detailed in this chapter, the empirical-collaborative method reaches beyond the observable to seek out elusive, nebulous, yet, nonetheless clinically relevant information
- Knowledge about Ben's personal, interpersonal, and family life helps explain his sense of emptiness and social detachment
- Ben's emotional state is driven by his unfulfilled interpersonal needs, reaching a crescendo in his emotional desperation

---

Clinical Illustration: Ben (4)

© The Author(s), under exclusive license to Springer Nature Switzerland AG 2023
S. A. Frankel et al., *Complexity in Health Care*,
https://doi.org/10.1007/978-3-031-14949-8_40

Unpacking clinical information is quite familiar to most of us. To understand a patient's presentation, we refer to books and journals, looking up pertinent information under familiar headings. It becomes difficult when there is a mixture of medical-psychiatric and psychological-social categories. Our method for unpacking the clinical complexity for a case follows, using Ben as an example.

The following description was initiated by Ben's psychotherapist. On first encounter, Ben was despondent. He was diagnosed with major depressive disorder, recurrent ICD-11 (F 32.1). Depressive disorder can be subdivided by its characteristics. Here are possible subcategories (Table 40.2).

Ben was further described as "immobilized, devoid of joy, unable to attend to his wife and daughters." There was no thought disorder evident. It seemed like a straightforward clinical situation. Not hard to understand. At least until you got to know Ben.

Let us start with the empirical, the observable. Psychiatric workups typically start there.

Ben was a rather handsome man whose personal habits reflected his Australian background. His restricted affect was observable as muted facial expression. With his boyish Paul McCartney "mop-top" haircut he reminded were reminiscent of musical figures from the 1980s. His speech was dotted with Australian variety British-isms such as "Mum" for mom; "mate" was injected frequently.

On first encounter, when his psychotherapist offered his hand to Ben, Ben immediately began to withdraw his. It would have been hard to tell from Ben's demeanor that he craved a relationship in which he could feel understood. You already know that Ben was smart, smart enough to find his way to Great Britain as a 19-year-old and prior to that create a phenomenally successful performing group in Australia, even while in secondary school. This level of aptitude was apparent any time you met and talked with him. Dapper, smart, successful as a youth, but abjectly depressed by age 40.

Our method mandates that we search for detail. The interviews with Ben are in part reproduced here. Family-genetic information helps. Ben had no siblings. According to him, both his parents were devoid of affect. His father who had been in the military was apparently a "gentle" human being but almost totally affectless. His mother was "nondescript almost nonexistent." Past high school, Ben saw no reason to remain in Australia since life there was so "bleak." Ben's father died when he was 32. No fanfare. Ben didn't even come home for the funeral. Apparently, his mother hardly reacted as well.

Table 40.2 Subcategories of major depressive disorder (ICD-11)

F33.1 Major depressive disorder, recurrent, moderate
F33.2 Major depressive disorder, recurrent severe without psychotic features
F33.3 Major depressive disorder, recurrent, severe with psychotic symptoms
F33.4 Major depressive disorder, recurrent, in remission
F33.8 Other recurrent depressive disorders
F33.9 Major depressive disorder, recurrent, unspecified

Regarding the collaborative piece, it was helpful for me to have a family member, a cousin, available to supply historical information. The dearth of information was apparently not due to superficial interviewing. Ben said he was not aware of any life events that might have personally affected him.

A life-changing fact did surface, however. After probing, Ben revealed that his past was contaminated by his having fathered a child out of wedlock. The pregnancy was the result of a "casual" but subsequently "haunting" affair in his early 20s. He provided money for the child's maintenance but "for some reason" always remained distant from the mother and child.

Ben's guess was that his "empty" early history and possibly his genetic background of depression afflicting both parents contributed to his own propensity for depression. One might infer that Ben was repeating his own experience of parental inadequacy in his lack of involvement with the child he fathered. In support of this development being a repetition of his early experience, I (SAF) found myself feeling oddly depressed as I wrote this passage. It was as if I had taken partial ownership of Ben's regret about having neglected this child.

By now you are probably beginning to become aware of a central paradox in this case. Ben was ostensibly devoid of emotion. Yet, he was able to create a spectacular performing group at age 15 and then move to a remarkable career as a computer programmer specializing in the creation of electronic music. Our method again mandates that we assiduously search for clues to resolve this paradox. Attention to Ben's past using the E-C method yielded striking, likely implicating, information that could be used to more deeply understand him.

Return to our progression using the E-C method: (1) Exhibit ("a") is the Guinness Book of Records, the single memorable purchase made by his parents during Ben's childhood. Remarkably enough, this acquisition appears to have been transformational for Ben, providing an imagined future that contrasted with his barren current environment. (2) Exhibit ("b") is that as an adult, on a visit to Australia, Ben contacted a family who had lived next door to him during his childhood. He had been given a tip by a relative that something important and out of the ordinary had happened during his childhood. What he found "shocked" him. Ben discovered that he had a sibling, a sister. She had been adopted out to an aunt. This event all occurred when Ben was a toddler. The shock was that this child, now an adult, was the mother of the child he fathered. She had been introduced to him as a cousin and nothing more about her identity was ever revealed to him.

Perhaps you can now begin to understand the aridness and confusion of Ben's childhood. The family's secrets around this subject had been totally buried. The truth about his sister and discussion about her had been sealed. In retrospect, everything in Ben's family had been organized around this event. Hopefully, you can now begin to see how deeply these buried truths must have affected Ben.

The issue is how to discover undisclosed features of a person's experience, especially when that person is unaware that these may be relevant to treatment. The clues may be discernable in the subject's demeanor and preferences but not understood by him or her as significant. For example, Ben had wanted nothing more than to "get away" from Australia, get away from school, and get away from conversation. Just get away. You could feel this when with him. But he rarely articulated these desires.

Emotional connection was hard for him to develop and sustain. And Ben felt it too. Meaning in his life proved elusive for him. Life was bleak, unpromising, a state of mind conflicting with his remarkable talents. To understand him, as you would need to take these attitudes (discouragement, disconnection, sense of purposelessness) seriously and mine them for meaning.

Another clue. Ben attached himself to his psychiatrist-psychotherapist as if he was "hanging on to life itself." Emotional desperation in the context of "nothingness." To respond appropriately, the treater would have to become absorbed by Ben's experience (as described earlier in this book) losing his/her sense of self in that interaction. Said differently, the clinician would need to allow him/herself to be taken in by the patient. From this state, the clinician can best understand what the patient wants to convey.

Retuning to Ben, how to understand his paralysis? Ben had all the qualities to be a great success. Everyone told him that. The professional society to which he belonged honored him repeatedly, lifting him to almost deity-like status. Remarkably, even when anticipating a packed hall, Ben saw no reason to prepare for his presentations. Ben's "Hall of Fame"-like stature was there in spades but he couldn't embrace it.

Was Ben depressed? Maybe, but the emotions seemed different from those of a typical depressive disorder. Ben expressed his despair in a book of sketches he published, a book with no words.

He disappeared from home episodically, and reminiscent of the song, "American Pie," he drove to a riverbank and just sat. Suicidal, yes, at least he thought a lot about suicide. No, in that his description about these moments was simply that they were "empty." He described his state of mind at these times as simply as "empty." The words of the song "drove my Chevy to the levy but the levy was dry" fit nicely [1].

So, who was this guy? What was the nature of his aridness? How would a clinician find out about his state of mind, a situation Ben called "emptiness" not "depression?" And that's what we have been after, a method for yielding a true picture of Ben's experience.

– Step "a" (empirical): record the information the patient provides, getting the data from the patient in his or her words so little is missing.
– Step "b": relate to the patient as a collaborator. "This is what I heard you say, tell me more.
– Step "c": clarify the ensuing dialogue. "I do not understand, can you help me?"

With Ben it might go as follows:

– SAF: "You say you feel dead inside, no emotion. But, you are here for something specific."
– Ben: "Right something human … something human. Do you understand?"

Let's sum up the yield. What can we infer about Ben and his inner life from this interaction? We start with his emotional "emptiness." Not only is Ben constricted. He is feeling dead. Nothing inside.

But there actually is a lot inside, just not utilized. According to others, he is brilliant and creative. Yet according to his own account, what he craves is human connection. His background is consistent with emotional bleakness, parents unable to provide an emotional connection.

It seems permissible to speculate about the psychological components of Ben's life and how they interrelate. Start with constriction, emotions not just overregulated but possibly obscure to him. Think of a toddler whose parents never provide feedback (in the child development literature called "affective attunement" and "mirroring"). In that situation, the child is emotionally stranded, little emotional input from other people.

So, now you have an example of the empirical-collaborative method and its potential yield. With the information, we have been able to glean Ben is no longer a nondescript human being. Not only can we begin to understand him, but we can empathize with him. Mental health treatment would potentially have initiated emotional expansiveness, emotion not yet built in.

Reference

1. Books LLC. Songs written by Don McLean: American Pie, Vincent, and I Love You So (L. L. C. Books & Books Group, Eds.). Books; 2010.

The Empirical-Collaborative Method and Its Fit with Clinical Complexity

41

Introduction

In this chapter, the cases of Seth and Andrew are used to identify and unravel ("deconstruct") the "#1", "#2", and "#3" variables encountered clinically. This process of deconstruction is intrinsic to the "empirical-collaborative method." Discussion in this chapter goes beyond the identification of salient variables and associated clinical information. Added is consideration of the strength and magnitude of contributing variables. We also reference the Value-Based Intermed Complexity Assessment Grid (VB-ICM-CAG). As previously mentioned, this clinical tool is used to unravel complex clinical situations.

Unpacking Complex Clinical Situations

What makes traditional methods for deconstructing the clinical field frequently so anemic, so likely to yield a false picture? Contributing variables may be missed or improperly emphasized or deemphasized.

Seth wanted desperately to repair the long-standing rift with his mother. He irrationally blamed himself for it. By now, she was bedridden from complications of cancer. She complained endlessly as she struggled with pain in her perineum. Her tendency to blame others was accentuated. The pressure on him was manifest through migraine headaches. These had previously been treated with sumatriptan but the treatment was losing its efficacy. Additionally, he was having trouble falling and staying asleep. He found it hard to work and was incessantly preoccupied with his mother's dissatisfaction.

His physician was of no help. She prescribed lorazepam 0.5 mg twice a day as needed and had increased it to 1 mg three times a day. He was relieved to have this

---

Clinical Illustrations: Seth (3) and Andrew

© The Author(s), under exclusive license to Springer Nature Switzerland AG 2023
S. A. Frankel et al., *Complexity in Health Care*,
https://doi.org/10.1007/978-3-031-14949-8_41

medication available to him but was sleepy throughout the day, making driving a risk. When queried about his emotional state, Seth could hardly respond. He did not think his now 82-year-old mother's illness was having an impact on him. He understood that his wife's anger at his mother and her disruptive intrusions was making his life stressful. There were also business problems, with several key clients threatening not to renew their contracts. Recounting the list, there were Seth's mother's new illness, her irritability, her ever-present threat to remove him from her will, his wife's quarrel with his mother, and his business problems. None of these factors were trivial.

But how to order these items in terms of their importance to Seth's health problems?

- According to Seth, the order was as follows: his wife's dissatisfaction with him and his anxiety about his mother reducing his share of her will. His business was suffering, but he believed that it was affecting his state of mind less than the other factors.
- Note that for another person, the list could have been quite different. For example, Seth's wife would put the discord with Seth's mother first on her list, and his wife was entirely indifferent to Seth's business problems. She said she loved Seth but was angry at him and was disinclined to help by accommodating his needs.
- His mother's physician, of course, had a different order of relevance, putting Seth's mother's medical condition first. Seth's personal physician who had limited time to devote to him was singularly interested in Seth's medical illnesses and in moving on to her next patient.

It is not hard to see why the empirical-collaborative method is an appropriate way of unpacking situations of this sort, and, in fact, virtually any complex clinical situation.

Apart from multimodal psychometric methods such as:

1. The Minnesota Multiphasic Personality Inventory (MMPI-2)
2. "Projective assessments" like the Rorschach test or its current incarnation
3. The R-PAS Performance Based Test

It is hard to think of other assessment techniques that would be as productive at deconstructing a complicated clinical situation.

OK. The next question for us to tackle has to do with magnitude. Our clinically based tool, "the empirical-collaborative method," allows us to deconstruct complicated clinical situations. However, we have no way of knowing how important each item is to outcome apart from using statistics, e.g., multiple regression analysis to ascertain the impact of each independent variable on outcome. We have already noted that individuals in a clinical situation, for example, Seth, his wife, his mother, and the involved physicians, are likely to rate the importance of individual items differently.

Andrew: Magnitudes of Contributing Factors

Andrew's personal situation was uneven. He was 45 and the father of two children. His animosity toward his own father was unbridled. His father's dissatisfaction with Andrew was equivalently raw. Financial problems plagued Andrew. His mother suffered from the long COVID-19 syndrome and was subject to dramatic flares of emotion. These often were exacerbated by emotional episodes.

How to judge the impact of individual factors (variables) in complex situations like this one? Are there standard methods for doing this? One could rate the impact of each contributing item such as Andrew's father's rage. But what would that factor be packaged with? For example, the simultaneous influence of Andrew's wife being out of work? We could attempt to quantify the personal impact of his father's contribution but taken alone that would be a simplification. These are components of the matrix of clinical factors making up Andrew's current experiential world. Each is semi-independent in its impact, but rarely experienced alone.

Formal Methods for Rating the Magnitudes of Components of a Clinical Situation

Let's return to Roger Kathol et al.'s previously described VB-ICM-CAG (see schematic diagram below). It consists of a thoughtfully constructed set of variables representing four clinical dimensions: medical, psychiatric, social, and care delivery. Each item offers four ratings for degree of urgency, and in most cases, a choice of time periods. Ratings are supported by online definitions (available through computer program) and clarifications. They are intended to be put into play by a case manager who uses the rated items to create a treatment plan. However, in the VB-ICM-CAG, there is little provision for the effect of interactions between variables and inclusion of variables that have limited clinical impact.

When clinically formulating Andrew's case, it would be tempting to leave out his distress at being reviled by his wife and father separately. His physician's focus would probably be on Andrew's obesity (not mentioned earlier) and prediabetic status. Andrew's personal distress is unlikely to be emphasized by her, and it would be most difficult to accurately predict how single contributing factors, e.g., his father's constant disapproval, might impact the success or failure of his treatment.

If we were to use a VB-ICM-CAG rating grid to make predictions, we might initially find it reassuring because of its detail and comprehensiveness (traversing four clinical dimensions). But the VB-ICM-CAG without case manager's notes would still not be a full rendering of clinical reality (Table 41.1).

Table 41.1 INTERMED–Complexity Assessment Grid (IM-CAG) (schematic view)

	Historical	Current state	(Future) vulnerability
Biological domain	1. Chronicity	1. Symptom severity/ impairment	Complications and life threat
	2. Diagnostic dilemma	2. Diagnostic/therapeutic challenge	
Psychological domain	1. Barriers to coping	1. Resistance to treatment	Mental health threat
	2. Mental health history	2. Mental health symptoms	
Social domain	1. Job and leisure	1. Residential stability	Social vulnerability
	2. Relationships	2. Social support	
Health system domain	1. Access to care	1. Getting needed services	Health system impediments
	2. Treatment experience	2. Coordination of care	

Using the Empirical-Collaborative Method to Arrive at a Paradigm Shift for Clinical Practice

42

Introduction

This chapter continues to elaborate our empirical-collaborative method. Deconstruction of the cases of Kamile and Erin using the empirical-collaborative method (E-C) revealed information that had been omitted or was not apparent on presentation. Kamile at first showed characteristics of a schizoid personality disorder. Further consideration using the E-C method revealed several incongruities including the discovery of a powerful desire for professional success. There were similar omissions in the case of Erin whose congenital defects were minimized by her family and not reported to medical practitioners. Neither Erin nor her family were aware of the profound emotional impact these defects were having on Erin.

Variety

We return to our cases with the objective of demonstrating how the E-C method can be used to unpack their complexity. If you look at the accompanying table, you will have a hard time finding commonalities in the clinical challenges presented by members of this group of patients. We have repeated the table here, this time including more clinical information about each patient. Some patients like Matthew (the boxer) are promising, perhaps clinically difficult but not complicated logistically. Others like Ben are steeped in travail and are unlikely to thrive under the best clinical circumstances.

Joining them is that as a group, they are so different one from another (heterogenous). This is precisely what one finds in clinical life. You may have a handful of "depressed" patients but they are likely to be very different one from

---

Clinical Illustrations: Kamile (3) and Erin

© The Author(s), under exclusive license to Springer Nature Switzerland AG 2023
S. A. Frankel et al., *Complexity in Health Care*,
https://doi.org/10.1007/978-3-031-14949-8_42

another when looked at closely. Your job is to decide what experience and equipment you need for treating each new patient. Complex cases, complex environments. Growing up in the Bronx was the same way. You never knew what you would find around the corner in the next neighborhood.

Please review this list again:

- Juliana (Seth's mother)—irascible, potentially withholds Seth's access to his inheritance
- Seth (software developer)—in conflict about loyalty to wife and mother
- Omar (Saudi Arabia)—theme of cheating or being cheated (cultural)
- Beth (diabetic woman)—terribly anxious about long-term use (contrast between her concerns and physician's)
- Jasmine (the woman from Yemen with schizophrenia)—paranoid in part culturally based
- Herb (polyarteritis nodosa)—secretive about being ill
- Nafi (unrequited love)—initially oppositional with doctor, proves his capability
- Maggie (elderly woman with vaginal cancer)—irascible but wise
- Ben (from Australia)—unremitting depression
- Londyn (normal early life, but increasingly depressed)—downward trajectory
- Jess (adopted twice)—originally progressing, now deteriorating (use of drugs and alcohol)
- Kamile (rule out schizoid personality disorder)—personally isolated at first
- "Mother" who commits suicide—unremitting depression
- Matthew (17-year-old boxer)—unreliable relationships, paradoxical respect by clinician

On a macroscopic level, most patients are accepting of their commonalities with others. However, on a microscopic level, we challenge you to come up with patients who want to be carbon copies of another person. Some patients are medically complicated, while others not. But all are complex when the "#1", "#2", "#2a", "#2b", "#3a", and "#3b" variables in each case are considered.

As clinicians, we do use similar tools for working with each case. We gather and methodically process all the data we can about the case using conventional diagnostic procedures. However, with anything short of the process we describe (the E-C method), what we think we know about each patient is an approximation, often a misrepresentation of that person.

Having lived for a while, you are undoubtedly aware that in "real life," complexities are paramount. For a patient to feel satisfied with the details of a case description of herself, she would have to feel distinguished from most other people, not "put into box." The empirical-collaborative method is our clinical tool for identifying and making selections based on these differences.

Return to Kamile. Factors contributing to her clinical diagnosis of schizoid personality disorder included, indifference to social norms and expectations, withdrawal from social activities, a preference for solitary activities including those

Table 42.1 Summarized from ICD-10, schizoid personality disorder includes:

- Choosing few activities that provide pleasure
- Limited capacity to express emotions
- Apparent indifference to praise or criticism
- Little interest in sexual experiences
- Prefers to be alone
- Preoccupation with fantasy life
- Lack of close friends
- Uninterested in prevailing social norms

based in fantasy. Summarized from ICD-10, schizoid personality disorder includes the following: (Table 42.1).

This designation fits well for a start. We could leave it at that, except that Kamile was atypical in ways. From the beginning, in contrast to her blunted affect, she seemed to devour the interpersonal part of psychotherapy, clamoring for more time with her psychotherapist. She quickly becomes attached to him and her primary care physician (PCP) as well.

Return to Erin

It may seem odd that Erin's pediatrician and parents did not report her medical condition to her psychiatrist and psychotherapist. But maybe not so odd. Omissions of this magnitude occur frequently in clinical work and often lead to misdiagnosis. The source is the subject's wish that medical problems disappear. Rejecting evidence adds a new kind of challenge to the case.

When I first met them at Erin's age 40, her parents had almost forgotten about the diagnosis she received at age 15. For that 25-year period, Erin's intimate life had been truncated, but her work life had not. She remained industrious and maintained a "cheerful" work demeanor. She became the mainstay of the family floral business. But all that mysteriously collapsed upon returning from visiting a male friend. The change in Erin was astonishing. No one could guess why this was happening. Erin rapidly grew ill-tempered, serially picking fights with her parents and siblings. She demanded that she receive her inheritance immediately.

There was no way to understand this dramatic change. Diagnostic speculations by her psychotherapist and parents, and then a psychiatric consultant, included (1) a "psychiatric (paranoid) breakdown," (2) a plot instigated by her Asian male friend to gain control of Erin's soon-to-be inherited wealth, and (3) Erin's medical limitations that were also raised as possible etiological explanations but not seriously considered until later.

The next (shocking) development occurred in a meeting with a lawyer, when Erin's sister's children were proposed for being included as heirs to the family's wealth. At that moment, Erin flared up. She screamed, "That money is mine… I've earned it… I deserve it. I can't have children and am entitled to this money." Erin's inability to have children and associated physical abnormalities were suddenly up front. Arriving at this point had required that other explanations be tried and exhausted.

In this case, the empirical-collaborative sequence consisted of a multiple step process for eliciting and screening information. A mixed deductive-inductive method followed by extensive interpersonal exploration was required to unpack this complex interpersonal situation. More specifically, this process included moving from a vague idea about developmental trauma to the emergence of a long-guarded secret about Erin's medical condition.

The Empirical-Collaborative Method and the Paradigm Shift, Further Illustrated

43

Introduction

Cardinal features of a case may be and often are obscure. Think again about Kamile: at age 14 she was highly inhibited, social development was delayed, and she had little or no interest in sex. And yet, in the end, there were clear indications that this wasn't the whole story. As in many cases, this lackluster candidate existed on an explosive store of hidden, often guarded, thoughts and opinions. The E-C method is designed to unpack a complex case like this one, revealing its clandestine features.

Kamile

To get a more complete picture of her, we will follow Kamile to age 30. How could one know what to expect as Kamile grew older? Refined assessment methods such as the VB-ICM-CAG when applied to a case like this should be helpful. The VB yields a "complexity score" that can inform us not just about the complexity of the case but also about which clinical information is likely to be most predictive of outcome.

How to unravel the patient's complexity and potential for progress? Can we rely on the E-C method to reveal the hidden clinical features? What can it tell us about the importance of individual aspects of the case, facts, participants, potential for twists and turns, planning?

Ben was about to give up, making suicide a real possibility. Kamile was a "deadbeat" ... little hope for progress. Erin was deteriorating (in her words, "defective"). And, yet, inexplicably Ben went on to attend to his daughters and join back with the wife he had labeled as "useless." Kamile ultimately found a "calling" as a scientist. And, shockingly, Erin ruthlessly (and sadly) sued her family for all their assets.

Clinical Illustration: Kamile (4)

© The Author(s), under exclusive license to Springer Nature Switzerland AG 2023
S. A. Frankel et al., *Complexity in Health Care*,
https://doi.org/10.1007/978-3-031-14949-8_43

So, how can we predict outcomes, especially those as unexpected as these were? Start with intuition. Clinicians rely heavily on intuition in the form of clinical judgment. Even if their work is "evidence-based," there is usually a "seat of the pants" aspect to their decisions.

Uh Oh, here we go again. What about mathematical justification and "confidence intervals" in statistics, the extent to which a prediction can be relied upon. When intuition is applied, these validated measures inevitably falter. Apart from empirical (real life) data, what you have with a clinical problem is at least in part contributed by inference.

It is interesting to note that virtually every clinical system requiring accuracy is in part speculative (based in approximation). Return to work as a clinician. As clinicians, we can hardly tolerate uncertainty in situations such as those involving life and death, cancer, heart problems, and domestic violence. However, do we have a choice?

Back to Kamile. Colorless, insisting on predictability. What she wanted was a life of absolute certainty: reliable parents, reliable friends, and reliable future. And she was irascible when these expectations could not be met. Introducing a goal without a predictable path for achieving it frequently enraged her. This level of imperfection would not have been tolerated in the almost "perfect" household in which she was raised? For greater clarity, let's try the E-C method. To do that with Kamile, we asked her questions, lots of them. And here is what we discovered.

Kamile's parents had delivered contradictory messages from early on. They represented themselves as strict and principled. Here is what Kamile discovered. Prior to Kamile's birth, her parents had been divorced and remarried. Kamile had once been told about the divorce but "forgot" about it and suppressed it. From that point (the point when she was informed about the divorce), Kamile progressively walled herself off socially, deciding that she simply did not like people who were different from those in her family. For safety, she buried herself in the adventure game, Dungeons and Dragons; her peak accomplishment was becoming a "dungeon master."

However, she couldn't fully avoid noticing that boys and sex were part of life. So, by age 24, she took an alternative path, this time involving "furries," animal figures that are eroticized and perfect for romantic and sexual fantasies. Of course, this development isolated her further since she had to work so hard at hiding these interests. She was referred for psychiatric treatment at grade 7. She had become isolated, began to suffer from panic attacks, and grew increasingly unpleasant in her relationships.

What is remarkable about this story is the efficiency with which Kamile hid her erotic interests. However, her attempts at deception progressively failed and became personally costly for Kamile and her parents.

Over the next several years, Kamile's Dungeons and Dragons friends went on to take jobs and attend college. Out of desperation and in response to family pressure, Kamile reluctantly agreed to attend a state college in Montana. What a disaster. The rustic atmosphere was opposite to anything Kamile had ever encountered. She soon stopped attending class and after two semesters was forced to withdraw from the school. Think of the contrast between Kamile's superior intellect as demonstrated earlier through neuropsychological testing and this outcome.

Hopefully, you can use this example to see the value of the E-C method for ferreting out hidden clinical information and detecting errors in reasoning. This process is best supported by clinical judgment bolstered by clinical instruments with good predictive ability (statistics) and repeated determinations of clinical progress. These determinations are best arrived at collaboratively. A key person in the collaboration is the patient, his or her willingness to ask hard questions and tolerate the unexpected and unpalatable.

Part XV

Understanding and Working with Clinical Complexity

[Part Introduction: Our current objective is to tie together all pieces of the book: our understanding of clinical complexity, how to manage it, the original model of clinical process, our revised paradigm, our method for validating our observations (the E-C method), our clinical method for engaging patients. Clinical work is first and foremost a human endeavor requiring flexibility, patience, and genuine empathy for the patient. We will not immediately return to the technical issue of statistical validation because that is reserved for a different portion of the book, separate from the clinical sections. Our goal is to be inclusive as we advocate for our revised and, in ways, new clinical paradigm.]

Excessive Certainty by the Clinician

44

Introduction

In this chapter, we review a case which called into question the clinician's (SAF) judgment and underscores the principle that a clinician needs to rely not only on research-based data for guidance but also on his or her own experience and clinical judgment.

Clinical Judgment: Its Virtues and Perils

The perils of exercising judgment freely within a professional context is likely to include clashing with the opinions of colleagues. The virtues may be peace with yourself, knowing you didn't make a pact with the devil by falsifying your opinions in conformity with a prevailing view.

Well, it's all well and good to be at "one with yourself". Good for the soul. But is it good for your patient? We would argue that when supported by credible data, usually it is.

Apart from hard data, verification in clinical work also comes from two subjective sources, yourself as clinician and your patient. Return now to mini-magnetic fields. These attract and repel, the polarity and strength of each field repeatedly changing. Human interaction is similarly unstable.

Back to a patient, this time Carol, and my clinical judgment as it evolved in her case. She was a complainer, but otherwise a seemingly well-intentioned 76-year-old woman whose husband had died 10 years earlier. Her new physician had only chart notes from her previous treatments available to him at the time of this consultation. He really hadn't had much time get to know her personally.

Clinical Illustration: Carol

© The Author(s), under exclusive license to Springer Nature Switzerland AG 2023
S. A. Frankel et al., *Complexity in Health Care*,
https://doi.org/10.1007/978-3-031-14949-8_44

I had been intermittently called in to consult about her case over a 2-year period. Apart from findings from physical examinations, routine blood work, a neurological examination (performed by a neurologist), and a recent CT and MRI of her brain, I also had a "feeling" for Carol (as a person) based on our multiple encounters. Anecdotal "evidence" included knowledge of how easily Carol could put her doctors off as she required extra attention for her emotional and medical needs. Nonetheless, I was aware that she had been correct about her diagnoses on important past occasions when her doctors were skeptical about her opinions. That had apparently been true when a now treated cancer was diagnosed 7 years earlier. Clearly, much of my input at the time of my current consultation relied on my past personal experience with this patient and the opinions of some of the other medical personnel involved in her case.

Carol reported the onset of excessive fatigue and balance problems starting about 6 months previously. These symptoms were not yet being taken seriously (were considered to be "functional") by her primary care physician, but she persisted in her insistence that they were "real" and disabling.

Now a leap one year into the future. One of Carol's current complaints, fatigue, had been superficially controlled by the time of my next visit with her, but her balance issues had worsened. Her symptoms seemed increasingly threatening. One fall causing a femoral fracture and she might not survive given the extent of her frailty.

At this point, there was a team of physicians involved in her care: an internist, a neurologist, a physiatrist, and an orthopedic foot and ankle specialist, as well as me a consulting psychiatrist. No abnormal laboratory or radiological studies beyond a brain ultrasound and brain MRI were revealing. The ultrasound and MRI showed dilated cerebral ventricles that had been noticed several years earlier and had been assumed to be congenital and nonprogressive. My clinical judgment at this point was to acknowledge my uncertainty about her diagnosis and wait.

The case was also sent to a physical therapist whose "go slow" wisdom and "meat and potatoes" recommendations ironically ended up being particularly helpful for identifying treatment measures that proved helpful for making a diagnosis. He recommended that Carol's condition be observed for a sustained period of time, at least until a definitive diagnosis could be established. During this period, as often happens when a case is on hold, a different feature of the patient's condition became prominent. Carol's lower legs and hamstring muscles were found to be intermittently spastic. This condition was causing her to shuffle as she walked. She avoided situations involving locomotion to protect herself against tripping and falling.

My (SAF) clinical sense was that her current symptoms were primarily medical and emphasized hamstring spasticity, but also included a likely psychiatric overlay. This opinion proved to be correct. The method of arriving at it was indeed inductive and collaborative, and was consolidated by involving each member of the treatment team.

In summary, Carol's presenting condition appeared to be irrefutably medical. While Carol evidenced severe anxiety, a primarily psychiatric etiology was ruled out. The most logical basis for her spasticity had been, of course, Parkinson's disease. But she had no tremor and her mobility pattern was not typical of Parkinson's.

The jury was and is still out. In sum, her nonspecific diagnosis was tentatively established as progressive neurodegenerative disease as yet unspecified.

Our current focus in this text, however, is on the use of clinical judgment and how that should come into play when diagnosing and treating a patient. In this case, Carol was my partial guide. Her judgment about her illness has proven to be reasonably accurate. She was clearly suffering, shocked by the rapid development of her balance problem, and made uneasy by the lack of clarity of her clinicians. She was also overwhelmed by the plethora of medical opinions offered to her. However, as a patient, she had little medical recourse other than to follow and rely upon the clinical judgments of her clinicians and press them to continually recheck their opinions.

Information accumulated. We had plenty of medical expertise available to us, but the most informative sources turned out to be the physical therapist, my clinical judgment, Carol's opinion about her illness, and the passage of time. My judgment was cumulative and partially relied on my familiarity with her case from our previous 2-year intermittent relationship.

A Retrospective

An implicit message here is about rigidly held views that become dogma. These certainly take their toll on unwitting students and clinicians who need to believe in the wisdom and indeed the integrity of "experts." Instead, it may be that what truly matters is the way these experiences of sticking with one's own opinions help us to become acquainted with ourselves (our biases and fallibility).

I believed I "knew" that Carol had a medical condition. But I was being dissuaded from fully believing it. The experience and the opinions of other involved physicians suggesting that her complaints were mainly "functional" were hard to resist. I intermittently "lost myself" as I worked on the case. Did I know anything more than what was obvious from the surface? Yes, I would have argued. But that view was unpopular.

Implications for Medicine

While not emphasized, in my experience with Carol, I was instinctively pulled to conform to the opinions of other physicians with whose opinions I differed. Their arguments were well defended and my differences with their opinions at times met with forceful opposition.

Freedom from Prescribed Truth

Physicians generally have extraordinarily high standards. Where I believe my colleagues went wrong in this case was simply in their skepticism about my clinical judgment. Where I went wrong, was in too easily accepting their point of view. The "takeaway?" Human considerations, flexibility, and real thought need to be repeat-edly renewed in medical work even when opposing opinions are compelling.

"Who am I?" is a cliché (a judgment rendered without much self-reflection), except when the challenge is deeply felt. The decision to "treat" another person and exercise clinical judgment is a profound undertaking. This level of involvement is hardly possible in the absence of self-reflection on the part of the clinician.

Achieving a "Real-Life" Understanding of a Case

45

Introduction

In this chapter, we bring back information from several of our cases in preparation for a more extensive discussion of an adapted use of "path analysis." As a technique, path analysis could be invoked to guide a clinician for working on a complex case involving multiple variables. Path analysis is a multivariate statistical method intended to identify correlations among multiple variables.

We are approaching a comprehensive understanding of the kind of information required for a "real-life" grasp of a case. This approach is the opposite to skimming over the patient's chart and inviting little follow-up. Certainly, Jennifer's just described interaction with the new internist who had only limited information about her would fall into that category. Also, relevant may be the contribution of unbidden situations to shaping treatment. For example, when the clinician becomes preoccupied because her daughter has to stay home from school with 102 °F fever and fails to pay close enough attention to details of the case.

Return to the classes of variables we have named to this point (Table 45.1).

Clinical Illustrations: Jennifer and Others

© The Author(s), under exclusive license to Springer Nature Switzerland AG 2023
S. A. Frankel et al., *Complexity in Health Care*,
https://doi.org/10.1007/978-3-031-14949-8_45

Table 45.1 Variables

"#1" variables	Variables that can be named, i.e., given an operational definition
"#2" variables	Variables, definitions for which are often difficult to establish, their manifestations multiple and fleeting. They are denotatively inexact. We have divided these into "#2a" habits of thought and behavior which may be culturally based and "#2b" which refer to motivation and emotion.
"#3" variables	Variables include those that constitute the building blocks of matter and experience.
"#3a" variables	Variables that are biological features of the clinical situation including (a) microscopic factors determining behavior and (b) genetic influences on behavior. These variables depend on the epigenome for existence and expression.
"#3b" variables	Variables that are poorly defined and may involve beliefs and thoughts originating in the mind of the subject

"Real-Life" Again

Neat collection, but we are momentarily struck by the fact that we have hashed over these categories with you earlier and fear we now risk boring you. We were moving along jauntily but could now be starting to lose vitality.

The problem we believe is in abstracting clinical observations. Even communicating our central idea, the paradigm shift, could become abstract and minimally informative. Ideas can be reduced to labels, e.g., diagnostic categories, and one's "sense" for the actual patient tends to get lost.

I almost must hear Carol's grating voice to authentically talk about the process of working with her. In brief, talking and thinking about a patient *in vitro*, as a specimen, provides incomplete information. *In vivo* (as a living organism), it regains its accuracy and vitality.

Before moving on, I (SAF) will again elaborate on the short-lived speaking blocks to which I alluded earlier. Phenomenologically, these experiences were like my frequent encounters with Jess when she tuned me out. "Cotton wool" surrounding me captures it. It was Kafkaesque, nothing to grab onto, nowhere to turn. Your mind freezes, and yet you must move forward since you are the writer/clinician. You grasp for something, anything to fill the void. The void here is that you do not really know what the patient needs or feels at that time. The temptation is to attribute your own ideas and feelings to the patient as if she were you.

With Jess this occurred, and it got worse and worse. She became more removed and inaccessible. As she faded, I felt progressively incompetent. I could have given her a diagnosis. "Major depressive disorder" would have been convenient. But it would have been an invention. More than likely, Jess had reached a point where psychotherapy had lost its promise. Alcohol must have seemed more attractive to her. Moving on in life (she was 26) was risky. Recall she had been adopted twice and each time she ended up with an adoptive "mother" who hated her.

It may be easier now to see why a static view of a patient is a trap. Relying on algorithms and diagnoses may be comforting but often is clinically misleading. It may also be falsely reassuring to have success with a patient and stop the treatment after initial success. In that case, you are not likely to be confronted with unwelcome developments.

To again see the circuitous path frequently taken by patients as we work with them, we return to Ben and his pessimism. As you may recall, Ben was an only child raised in emotional poverty. He left home as early as possible and found his way to England at age 19 where he started his career developing computer software and applying it broadly. Remarkably talented, he never could get excited about anything. Several medications were tried without any ongoing improvement in his mood and outlook. On several occasions, he was on the verge of suicide. It has been 2 years since last reporting to you about his progress.

Ben quit his job about a year after the last report about him. He had been a partner in a very successful company of four people, all outstanding designers. But Ben who was never satisfied with the mundane was unhappy in this commercially focused job. So, one day (in collaboration with his therapist), he quit it. The decision seemed catastrophic but the result nothing short of monumental. In Ben's words, "my sanity was restored."

Jennifer's life took an equally surprising turn. As her cancer progressed, she paradoxically became more civil. Everyone warned Jennifer that her judgmental surgeon would likely lose patience with her and limit his availability. However, remarkably, the opposite occurred. The surgeon apparently began to communicate respect for Jennifer. This change was seemingly based on her dogged commitment to her cancer treatments. She required multiple operations and chemotherapy and experienced unrelenting pain after her cancer spread. The "spoiled" Jennifer proved herself and earned (as he told her) the surgeon's highest praise.

As I write, I am no longer searching for a fresh clinical focus. Vitality was reinfused by our talking about the "real-life" Ben and Jennifer. Their clinical needs and determination remained fresh and challenging. It was me who had become bogged down insisting on looking for the familiar rather recognizing the unexpected.

Part XVI

Synthesis, Path Analysis

[Part Introduction: Path analysis was introduced in Part III, Chapter 4. It involves an examination of connections between and among variables, together with positing causal relationships. Our adaptation of path analysis (termed a "clinical path diagram") for use with individual complex clinical situations is novel. By doing this we take single clinical situations involving multiple variables and schematize them. In this part, we have attempted to do this with one of our cases, Jennifer, an elderly woman with multiple general medical and psychiatric illnesses.]

Use of Path Analysis to Map Out Complex Clinical Situations

46

Introduction

In this chapter, the complex clinical history of Jennifer is reviewed with the help of the empirical-collaborative method for exposing unappreciated variables. A hypothesized model of Jennifer's interaction patterns and causal relationships associated with the case are then formalized as a "path diagram." In the next chapter, we will use an adaptation of this statistical technique (path analysis) to achieve this end. "Path analysis" will allow us to view a complex case in composite, with all of its component parts and their clinical influence, considered.

Jennifer's Current Clinical Status

Jennifer is a tough case, each factor in her history influencing and modifying the others. We have tried to pay attention to as many of these often incongruent areas as we are aware of. And the outcome? Here it is. The source of each component is at least somewhat ambiguous.

Jennifer's traits on outcome:

- Tenacity: Jennifer has become tougher, and more resilient.
- Her cancer is in remission.
- She has colostomy and nephrostomy tubes that are personally troublesome. Jennifer is nicer. She is no longer butting heads with her adult children. She is more patient with her providers having finally established a fine relationship with her surgeon.
- Jennifer still exudes anxiety.

Here you can see the E-C method at work. We started with multiple "lumps of clay," a messy landscape consisting of symptoms, practitioners, and personal

S. A. Frankel et al., *Complexity in Health Care*,
https://doi.org/10.1007/978-3-031-14949-8_46

resources. Once we could get to work, parts separated and congealed, reshaping one another. Jennifer's resilience was tested. So was her clinician's capacity to both understand her medical condition and personal needs. Without Jennifer's continual input communicating her fears, and finally her wisdom, we would have quite a different clinical picture. It contrasts with that of a sick old lady. We challenge you to tell us which factors were most important in creating the temporary outcome we are now living with. That, dear reader, is the beauty of our adapted version of factor analysis (see next chapter).

Honestly, if you put yourself in the shoes of her surgeon, oncologist, or psychiatrist, would you collectively have the expertise to create the treatment we have described? Recall the major contributions of encouragement, support, and empathy. Truly a "witch's brew."

Back to implicated and proposed variables. "#1" variables are vaginal bleeding in an elderly woman, as well as fatigue and gait disturbance which needed to be confirmed. Side effects of tamoxifen could be implicated at this level. A key "#2" variable is severe anxiety which to some extent could lead to her fatigue and balance complaints. "#3" variables are biological factors associated with her cancer and requiring chemotherapy.

Return to the internist. He not only may have missed her diagnosis by not recognizing the extent and potential complications of her anxiety, but he also never considered diagnosing a neurological condition.

This type of clinical situation is more common than may be appreciated. Bring in the empirical-collaborative method. What if the physician in charge had done the following? (1) collaboratively checked with Jennifer's oncologist and family to see how prone she had previously been to develop anxiety-based symptoms and whether her medical symptoms at those times proved to be "functional"; (2) inductively unpacked her current symptoms to create a comprehensive differential diagnosis; (3) taken into consideration that in addition to her hypochondriacal tendencies, she was actually quite resilient and that symptoms she previously reported had generally been indicative of medical disease; and (4) waited until appropriate diagnostic evaluations could be assembled before formulating a management plan. Through speaking to her past primary care physician and after carefully studying her medical record, he would have discovered that for a while multiple sclerosis had been entertained to explain her intermittent episodes of fatigue, with balance problems.

A comprehensive evaluation might have included a detailed clinical history and physical and neurological examinations. Since multiple sclerosis (her gait disturbance) could be considered, he might order a lumbar puncture (particularly to look for oligoclonal [IgG] bands) and a brain and spinal cord MRI to look for areas of demyelination and tested for evoked potentials. Note that manifestations of MS are highly variable. Among the arguments against MS in this case is that the typical MS patient presents in early adulthood with distinct but variable and often fleeting episodes of CNS dysfunction often manifest as spastic paraparesis or cerebellar ataxia.

Important here is that medical diagnoses and treatment recommendations are both variable and fallible. These uncertainties depend on not only the patient's medical condition but also his or her emotional state and habitual tendencies. Physician certainty has no abiding place in making these determinations. False positives and negatives in physician judgment are common.

Clinical Judgment, Revisited

We now go back to clinical judgment, what is it and how certain a clinician can be about using it to make clinical choices?

Here are some of the assessment and treatment parameters that would be relevant for Jennifer's workup:

- The clinician's experience with the clinical issues case at hand.
- Information from technical/medical literature, history, and examination findings.
- Formal assessment/laboratory test data.
- Other involved professionals influencing the clinician's impressions and opinions; those supporting a physician's excessive pride could be an example.
- Patient nonacceptance of the clinical findings as well as alternative hypotheses introduced by the patient and any other member of the treatment team.

Prevailing methods (e.g., standards of care) often have a strong, and at times misleading, influence on practice behavior. These norms are hard and sometimes impossible to challenge and may improperly skew the clinical work. Thomas Kuhn's work on the difficulty of achieving a paradigm shift in science speaks forcefully about this issue [1].

Clinical Judgment

It is strange that from the start, I had such a strong opinion that Jennifer's derangement was medical, possibly something serious. In my mind, her symptoms couldn't just be the result of somatization. Granted that fatigue and gait disturbance may not be any more specific than symptoms associated with the "phantom" physically debilitation state called chronic fatigue syndrome (myalgic encephalitis). Apart from relatively specific diagnostic assessments such as lumber puncture and MRI (the specificity of which is reassuring but still not absolute), what we must rely on is Jennifer's reporting and the course of her symptoms. You need a cooperative patient (as a contrast, multiple sclerosis patients tend to be highly emotional) to be able to rule out a biological etiology from one that is triggered and mimicked by emotions.

This reasoning might make us more sympathetic with Jennifer's overly confident new internist, except that he was so cavalier in his approach to his new patient. So, apart from diagnostic tests, how could he and other clinicians be sure they get it right? However, complex clinical situations are rarely entirely straightforward since they encompass so much detail. But that also is their beauty. Imagine a clinical world that is devoid of nuance and mystery. So, at times, clinical judgment often may be our most reliable ally when doing clinical work.

At this point in this case, my opinion was that Jennifer was a little erratic. A fussy old lady used to being pampered by her doctors. Her internist might have been justified in being a bit fed up with her. Certainly, I was. After all her call came on my Saturday as well as his. But then the lab results began to become available. There was something more here. Her cerebrospinal fluid (CSF) was purulent. The case moved from yellow alert to red alert. Certainly, Jennifer's internist had gotten it wrong, but I also didn't anticipate this finding. For both of us, our clinical judgment was off base.

The clinician needs to be constantly engaged in a thought process in which patient variables together with intuition and hypothesis are considered. In the following chapter, prior discussion of interacting variables and path analysis is formalized to create a case formulation and treatment plan incorporating all the information we have collected about Jennifer.

Reference

1. Kuhn TS. The structure of scientific revolutions (50th ed.). University of Chicago Press. 2012.

Mapping Out Jennifer's Case, Using a Path Diagram to Schematically Represent a Complex Case

47

Introduction

In this chapter, the statistical method called "path analysis" is reviewed together with its analogue, the clinical "path diagram." In "path analysis," variable information about a case, e.g., information about Jennifer, is identified by lines connected to geometric symbols (e.g., rectangles), that, for example, may convey estimated strength of association, hypothesized causation, and amenability to selected treatment modalities. The result is a diagram that with minimal perusal provides the clinician an immediate "snapshot" of the patient's complexity and the priorities for treatment. Both the empirical-collaborative method and path analysis are useful for unpacking clinically unpacking and mapping out complex situations, exposing their component parts.

The procedures for constructing a clinical path diagram will be described and demonstrated with an actual path diagram, and we illustrate techniques for working with multiple correlated data points. Similar techniques each with approximately the same objectives include "path analysis," "factor analysis," and "structural equation modeling." We will restrict our discussion arbitrarily to "path analysis" and its ability to represent a complex clinical situation using annotated diagrams. The identity (linear relationship) between variables is determined and represented in each case by a "correlation coefficient." Variables when grouped together are called "factors." Manipulating these entities statistically is usually reserved for large collections of data that need to be analyzed by computer. However, we believe that the principles of this method can be usefully applied in unpacking and mapping out complex clinical situations that like our cases are comprised of smaller numbers of variables.

© The Author(s), under exclusive license to Springer Nature Switzerland AG 2023
S. A. Frankel et al., *Complexity in Health Care*,
https://doi.org/10.1007/978-3-031-14949-8_47

Path Analysis, Jennifer

Jennifer, 79 years old, was again our patient. She had a new internist. She had experienced uncharacteristic fatigue and unsteadiness of gait for 2 weeks. She also had intermittent vaginal bleeding. Her new internist was not given to admitting mistakes. He was proud of his skill and reputation, perhaps too proud. His patients tended to be well to do and prominent. He saw them at parties and regaled them with self-aggrandizing tributes to his uniqueness as a physician. He had a concierge practice, meaning that by contract he was committed to being available whenever his patients needed him. In this incident, Jennifer was in trouble. It was a Saturday morning. As she had been instructed to do, Jennifer called her new physician on his private cell phone but by afternoon he had not called back. Another physician was urgently called in to consult.

When her new internist finally was reached on Sunday morning, he apologized for not being immediately available and after hearing about Jennifer's symptoms offered consoling remarks. He was "sure" Jennifer would be "OK." He added that most likely there was nothing to worry about. The vaginal bleeding could be a side effect of tamoxifen, a medication she had taken for 3 years following treatment of breast cancer. Since he was not the specialist in charge of her cancer care, he would have to hand that issue off to her oncologist. He would, nonetheless, keep his eye on her blood loss. End of story. According to him, in addition to the bleeding, her fatigue and balance problems were probably due to aging, not likely to blood loss. He never considered a neurological condition. He would order some routine laboratory tests and she should go to the laboratory on Monday.

Notice this physician's confidence. He had a potentially serious medical situation on his hands (after all Jennifer had been treated for cancer) and yet he was quick to diagnose. He had taken only a short history over the phone and had no laboratory studies to back up his "off the cuff" assertions. Jennifer tended to be cantankerous, always critical of others. She was incessantly worried about her health, a tendency that raised suspicions that her complaints of fatigue and "balance problems" might be "functional."

A "clinical path diagram" for this case study is presented below. This approach is adapted from the work of Haynes et al. [1].

Based upon clinical judgment and insight, the arrows represent possible causal variables that influence the two main variables labeled in yellow. Also of note is a line with two arrowheads, representing a bidirectional causal relationship. Hypothesized strength of variables is in red. Circles and spheres represent medical issues; squares and rectangles represent psychological variables. Within certain of these geometric forms is hypothesized modifiability of the variables, and if viable, evidence-based procedures for accomplishing such modifications.

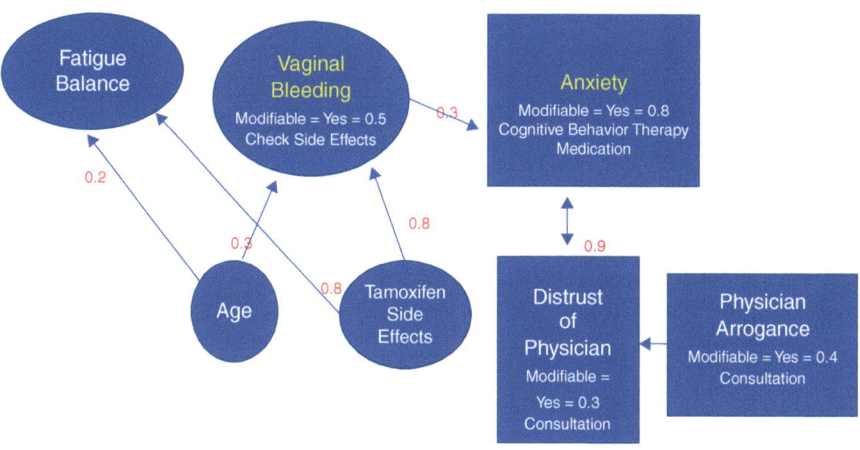

Diagram Definitions

1. Importance of behavior problem or medical problem: in yellow
2. Strength of causal relationship: 0–1 (same as correlation coefficient): in red
3. Estimated modifiability of psychological or medical problem: 0.2 = minimal; 0.4 = moderate; 0.8 = very high
4. Circles = medical or physical problems
5. Squares or rectangles = psychological problems
6. Lines with single arrowheads = hypothesized causal relationships. In red are numbers indicating hypothesized strength of the causal relationship
7. Lines with two arrowheads = reciprocal or bidirectional causal relationship

    With reference to the diagram above, the variables "vaginal bleeding" and "anxiety" are the important focal objects of treatment; hence, they are both listed in yellow. The two variables that are assumed to influence vaginal bleeding are age and the possible adverse effects of tamoxifen. The effect of age is posited to be weak (correlation in red of 0.3), whereas the side effect of tamoxifen is strong (correlation of 0.8). Within the circular geometric form for vaginal bleeding is a numerical estimate of modifiability. In this matter, it equals (0.5). The subjective estimate of the treating professional is that the problem has a moderate to high chance of being corrected and that the effect of tamoxifen is the likely culprit. The bleeding probably contributes to the patient's anxiety but to a minor degree (0.3) compared to the impact of "distrust of physician with reference to distrust of new internist" (0.9). Moreover, the relationship between Jennifer's anxiety and distrust of her new physician is reciprocal, as illustrated by the line with two arrowheads, i.e., it is shared by the consulting physician who is uncomfortable with Jennifer. Within the anxiety sphere, Jennifer's anxiety is hypothesized to be treatment responsive (0.8) to a combination of medication and cognitive behavioral therapy. Based on contacts with the new internist, the consulting clinician (Jennifer's original internist) posits that arrogance contributes to Jennifer's distrust but is not certain to what degree. He is willing to consult with the new internist but is not encouraged that consultation will be effective (modifiability = 0.3).

The information from the path diagram *differs from that of the narrative description*. The path diagram provides a compendium, a list of variables and estimates of their effect on Jennifer and the extent to which they interact. The narrative is detailed to a degree that a schematic diagram cannot be substituted. In effect, it consists of facts about the patient and instructions about what kind of actions should be taken for each of the patient's medical-psychiatric complaints. It is essentially an algorithm providing detailed instruction for action. But neither is complete. Both leave out important pieces of the patient's "real" condition.

Considered carefully both types of representation contribute to a clinician's understanding of a case. The path diagram is more in keeping with the practical, heuristic bias of contemporary medicine. The case illustration introduces nuances that contribute to understanding the patient in his or her full complexity. Both have their place when conducting clinical work, the path diagram approach being more reductive and convenient, as with all heuristic approaches.

Reference

1. Haynes SN, O'Brien WH, Godoy A. A proposed model for the psychometric evaluation of clinical case formulations with quantified causal diagrams. Psychol Assess. 2020;32(6):541–52. https://doi.org/10.1037/pas0000811.

Part XVII

Conclusion, Clinching the Paradigm Shift

[Part Introduction: In this part of the book, we will complete our shift to a revised clinical paradigm emphasizing the complexity and subjectivity of both patient and practitioner. In the first chapter of this part of the book, clinical complexity involved complications in my interaction with an attractive, ingratiating patient, Michael. He was hiding his legal troubles. From here this part of the book moves to didactic chapters describing complexity introduced by a clinical technique emphasizing abductive (creative) reasoning.]

Slowly Emerging Details

48

Introduction

In this chapter, we will continue our shift to a revised clinical paradigm that significantly includes the subjectivity of both patient and practitioner. In the chapter, clinical "failure" in SAF's case of Michael is discussed. In this situation, his misjudgment caused SAF to obsess about his possible misguided personal motives in accepting the case. Some approaches to avoid therapeutic outcomes such as this one, including through the use of the empirical-collaborative approach, are discussed.

Complexity in this case involved an attractive, ingratiating patient, Michael, who was attempting to keep his legal difficulties private. Complexity included (1) Michael's potential dishonesty about his motives for seeking treatment and his desire to hide his legal difficulties from his clinician, (2) SAF seeking consultation from a colleague after realizing he had violated his professional standards by being willing to accept a patient who was already in the partial care of another psychiatrist, and (3) SAF's excessive preoccupation with his clinical "failures" with this patient.

Clinical Illustration: Michael

Michael, a 60-year-old lawyer who told me that he had failed in nine other psychiatric treatments, was referred to me for a "consultation" and then treatment. According to Michael, no one had been able to understand or find a fix for his psychiatric problems. I was to be the last practitioner to try and likely fail. We carried on with our work for several months. And then without notice, it collapsed, Michael cancelling our "final" session.

Clinical Illustration: Michael

The failure was painful for me (SAF). So, painful that I inexplicably obsessed about it for weeks. I carried a vague sense of failure that generalized and affected my work. (I have had my share of failures over the past 40 years and expect them to occur occasionally, but this was unexplainably more difficult for me.) At first, I expected Michael to call back, repeatedly checking my phone and email. But he apparently meant it when he said he said he had decided that I could not help him and wanted nothing more to do with me. As a psychiatrist, you cannot please everyone and in fact should not expect to. Each patient, each case, is different. Often failure is not predictable. But my reaction to this failure was uncanny. Something had truly gone wrong. Something outside of my comprehension. Perhaps something fundamentally associated with my self-image had been challenged. He had read one of my books and said he had been strongly attracted to my ideas.

In retrospect, I had missed something, and it was substantial. Michael was "a charmer," always ready with incisive observations. Apparently, I had been convinced into believing that this case might be a perfect one for me. I could be the magician who performed the right trick. Yet I failed and was unable to anticipate the failure. Michael's request for help seemed earnest enough. He said he needed "help" and he believed that I was just the person who could provide it. I managed not to think about the nine psychiatrists (no exaggeration) who had preceded me. I also managed not to notice that I hadn't followed the rigorous sequence I usually stick to for gathering information at the beginning of a treatment. Not a good way to start a new treatment, and totally unnoticed by me since at the time I puzzlingly felt quite comfortable with my behavior.

More Information

In the past, Michael had managed to convince surgeons that he needed joint replacements when there were no surgical indications for these. Since I wasn't involved in these episodes, I cannot vouch for the capability of the recruited surgeons. I am certain that the need for these surgeries was never substantiated. I was able to recover this information retrospectively by re-examining Michael's medical record. You are probably aware that the situation being described, a patient obtaining surgeries for factitious disorder, is likely to be an example of Munchausen syndrome.

The point here is that details that are overlooked may matter a great deal in evaluating a clinical situation. But obtaining this new information about Michael's previous surgical misadventures did not decrease my sense of failure. It didn't seem to matter how much information I had about Michael's unorthodox medical-psychiatric behavior. Knowing how difficult it may be to examine one's own behavior I finally decided to speak to my psychologist friend Aaron. He surprised me by asking why I accepted the case when I knew that another psychiatrist was already involved. I struggled and confessed that I had been flattered by Michael's excitement after his reading about my clinical ideas. Part way into the conversation with Aaron, I began to freeze. It occurred to me that since Michael was a lawyer, he could be angling to expose my flaws, perhaps with a litigious motive. But Michael seemed so thoughtful and intelligent. He had seemed like the ideal case to fill an open slot in my COVID-19 beleaguered practice.

But how possible is it for a physician working on the fly to apply this degree of vigilance? On the other hand, how can he or she avoid it? As with Michael's knee replacements and other surgeries, without this degree of scrutiny, a physician could be treating a nonexistent condition. But, how then to ferret out the "truth?" I sought out his past medical records. I needed more information about these treatment failures and about the remarkable impact on me of his abrupt departure from our treatment.

I am loath to admit it, but the bottom line in explaining the degree of my posttreatment consternation appears to be my shame about my own desire to have a new case and my attendant lack of discrimination in evaluating his medical history. Up to this point, I have been placing responsibility on Michael, his idiosyncrasies and his tendency to cook up medical-surgical disorders. My painful discovery came because of my review of this case with Aaron. Usually, I am quite articulate about clinical matters but suddenly as I presented the case to him, I found myself becoming inarticulate. I faltered as I attempted to describe the case. I knew the facts but could not articulate them.

Aaron caught on quickly. "Why did you take the case, Steve?" I blushed, "well, it was a good case, interesting and worthwhile." "But what about the other psychiatrist involved?" This was a Raskolnikov moment, my own version of a "Crime and Punishment" scenario (Dostoyevsky, F. (2001). Crime And Punishment. Signet Classics). In this case, my speaking with Aaron invited a confrontation and engendered self-scrutiny like that of the E-C method.

It seems peculiar that this incident had such a profound effect on me. And yet I wonder. What if my clinical work could repeatedly but subtly be affected by similar oversights? I was quite proficient at recognizing Michael's flaws and personally citing these to explain my failure. In fact, I now recall Michael's lament that "none of you psychiatrists ever *really* apologize for your errors." Of course, I had no idea what he meant at that time. At first, I was quite "clear" about my earnestness in agreeing to treat Michael and my lack of culpability.

The "Takeaways"

We are rarely as pure as our intentions will us to be. Seriously, as I entered this case, I believed I was "as clean as the driven snow." As I exited, I became aware of the extent to which I had become sullied. During this process, I had no idea that I was compromising myself. My alter ego, the one that kept me from being articulate with Aaron, could attest to that. Am I a big-time sinner? No. Am I a sinner? Yes. Could I have caught myself? Maybe. But in this case, I needed help. Again, the point is that the details (comprising the complexity of the situation) matter. Had I been alert for these and willing to take them in, I believe I would have done a better job screening Michael and perhaps avoided misdiagnosis.

An Aside

Back to clinical practice. We have discussed personal measures for recognizing and dealing with the medical professional's personal failings, particularly those of physicians. Common failings may include excessive restriction of personal involvement with patients, suppressing emotions, and "doctor-like" authority manifest as aloofness as was the case with the physician described in Jennifer's case.

The likely outcome in Michael's case? You can answer that for yourself. The following are partial remedies given that as a physician the time you can spend with a patient is necessarily so limited, that there is so much distracting paperwork, and that reimbursement for services is often so paltry. These include adopting a collaborative team-focused approach emphasizing allied medical professionals who share responsibility for the clinical and at times the administrative work. Each patient is discussed at regular (usually weekly) team meetings and followed serially. When working in a community setting, it is often advantageous to see the patient in a place with which he or she is familiar and with familiar providers.

Surprise Ending

But none of the above will suffice for the painstaking exploration (including rigorous record review and interviews) required for working with patients like Michael. To do this, details truly mattered. How else can one pick out the hidden points of real significance for understanding the patient and case? With Michael had I persisted in trying to treat him and done so meticulously, I would ultimately have discovered a pattern of amphetamine misuse that was remarkably well disguised through his pursuit of medical care. His multiple treatment failures could have been a tip off. Earlier recognition of his psychopathy would have opened an entirely different view of Michael and the case.

This clinical situation called for consultation with a colleague and harsh self-reflection for the clinician.

Giving Up One's Assumptions in Pursuit of a Paradigm Shift

49

Introduction

Adopting new ways of thinking requires detachment from entrenched thoughts and habits. Achieving this end may involve a substantial paradigm shift for a practitioner. This creative process may include (a) new variable classifications, (b) use of statistical-type thinking (formal statistical thinking and modifications thereof), (c) abductive reasoning, and (d) a unique treatment relationship that may involve expansive experiences such as "awe."

Our goal in this book has been to identify a paradigm for clinical work that improves its accuracy and scope. Our model includes, and as pertinent, emphasizes variables that are often omitted and/or undervalued in clinical work. A crazy, complicated undertaking no doubt, but essential for clinical accuracy. After all, through shortcuts (heuristics, including summarizing through diagnostic categories and algorithms), one is likely to leave out details that matter and in effect falsify, creating a caricature of the patient.

Barriers to Change

Clinicians use and often "overlearn" skills consistent with the paradigms that were dominant in their training and practice. It seems axiomatic that clinicians would be hesitant to shift to a different way of seeing and working clinically.

The Semmelweis reflex, previously discussed, illustrates how practitioners may have difficulty shifting from an established way of thinking to another approach, even if the new approach is demonstrably more effective. The recommended behavior change in this instance was simply to wash one's hands before examining a patient. The change in thinking was accepting that invisible microbes can be transmitted to a patient via unwashed hands. This modification was originally incomprehensible for many physicians and stringently resisted.

Foundation for a Paradigm Shift

Procedures based on dominant (accepted) clinical paradigms may not produce effective results. We discovered (often to our discomfort) that to be effective with certain patients, our thinking had to change. There are dimensions of the clinical situation and a plethora of interacting clinical variables that we had not even contemplated as relevant. Our existing paradigm was too simple. Our thinking about patients had to be upgraded to a different paradigm with a greater array of clinical possibilities, i.e., in effect paralleling clinical complexity. This awareness was the beginning of the "paradigm shift" that led to writing this book.

Components of our shift, revising preexisting clinical formulations of clinical complexity.

1. *Variable classification.* As discussed, our paradigm shift goes beyond inclusion of traditional clinical variables and includes previously ignored or undervalued variables as well as the product of their interactions. In this book, we have attempted to classify variables in groups as "#1", "#2", "#2 subtypes", "#3a" and "#3b". Briefly, this classification is as follows: "#1" variables are clearly defined and particularly amenable to quantification; "#2" variables tend to be vague, not clearly defined and often amorphous; "#3a" may be components of an entity that has been named but is not directly observable (e.g. is biological, microscopic); and "#3b" are phenomenon that may only exist in the mind of either or both of the treatment participants. The variables we name may be characterized by their effects on other clinical phenomena in the same way that a magnetic field can be identified by its effects on ferromagnetic objects.

   The variables on which we focus have in part been chosen to expand clinicians' thinking about factors that have been deemphasized traditionally. We have previously discussed variable interactions and presented a diagrammatic approach (factor analysis) for representing complex interacting patient variables.

2. *Idiographic statistical thinking.* The clinician works with data gathered directly from the patient through interviews and test data. We have reviewed methods of measurement and data gathering and have urged readers to search nomothetic data sources. Again, nomothetic refers to research on groups of participants yielding summary statistics found in scientific writings. "Factor analysis", "path analysis", and structural equation modeling are statistical methods that mathematically identify common elements (correlations) among several, perhaps many, variables measured across numerous, at times thousands of, participants. This statistical method is impractical for rigorous use with individual patients, but the clinician can use principles of factor analysis to assist clinical thinking by informally discerning correlations among groups of variables. In that way, principles of path analysis, factor analysis, and structural equation modeling could be used informally as a way of thinking about more inclusive complex clinical situations.

3. *Abductive reasoning and patient collaboration.* We have discussed the scientific method as a major source of truth (validation) and have reviewed

the inductive and deductive processes typically used by scientists. In the paradigm shift, we go beyond inductive and deductive reasoning and advocate abductive thought processes (Chapter 15). Abductive thinking involves formulating explanatory hypotheses that can be explored in what we call an "empirical-collaborative" manner with the patient. The result is for parties to arrive at tentative conclusions about which revised hypotheses can be eliminated and those that should be pursued.

4. *A unique psychiatric relationship.* The paradigm shift we describe involves augmentation of the clinician-patient relationship. In our experience, a key to therapeutic progress involves clinician humility communicating the clinician's appreciation of the patient's personal (subjective) reality. As well, there is a distinct shift in focus from the clinician's humanity to that of both partners. This relationship may not sound much different than a traditional therapeutic bond. But, in our experience when achieved, this shift may lead to a dramatic change in perspective for both the clinician and patient, that is, an enhanced ability to comprehend the subjective experience of the other.

The following analogy may help to clarify the perspective alluded to. One of us (ST) has interacted with astronomers and physicists and observed how they "lose themselves" as they contemplate the vastness of space/time and the complexities of the interacting components within molecular fields. Added is the challenge of explaining the "spooky" (Einstein's word) world of quantum physics. They often use the word "awe" to describe encounters with the immense and far-reaching intricacies of what they observe. Importantly, this awe experience appears to have facilitated their capacity for creative observation, hypothesis formulation, and thought.

Similarly, in clinical situations as we have struggled to take in the equivalent vastness of a patient's subjective reality, we have had the profound experience of immersing ourselves in the awareness of the other's internal world. Subsequently, we discovered that investigators from several disciplines (e.g., physics, psychology, neuroscience) have labeled this experience "awe." The research on "awe" from the physical sciences seem to converge with that on "interpersonal awe."

Interpersonal Awe

Previously (Chapter 6), we discussed "awe" as a part of our paradigm shift or at least a metaphor that may facilitate the understanding of our recommendation for shifting therapeutic paradigms. This designation includes the neurological, physiological, and psychological aspects of the awe experience. Earlier we emphasized that awe is a complicated but profound emotional and cognitive experience. Awe was described by scientists as they contemplated the telescopic vastness of the universe and the prodigious shift in appreciation of the microscopic features of physical reality. Words such as "astonishment" and "wonder" are often used to describe one's personal experience of awe. A sense of awe can be engendered by the actions and information gleaned about the dynamic complexity of our fellow human beings. This experience is termed "interpersonal awe."

Although awe is usually engendered by overwhelming positive characteristics, it can also be evoked by stunning negative aspects of the physical world or personal attributes of fellow beings. The astrophysicist, for example, can be astonished with the expansion of the universe while simultaneously being apprehensive that the universe will expand until it ceases to exist. At times, interpersonal awe may also include astonishment and wonder based on horror about an individual. As mentioned earlier, one of us (ST) has worked with persons who have performed remarkable antisocial acts. The vast complexity of interacting genetic and environmental variables that produced someone capable of exterminating 42 persons in 13 states was indeed astonishing (serial killer Thomas Eugene Creech) and engendered what might be termed a negative sense of awe.

We suggest that "interpersonal awe" may also describe the therapeutic bond resulting from the paradigm shift we have described. The experience can be analogous to seeing microbes when first looking through a microscope. By instigating an experience of interpersonal awe, a clinician may activate fluency, flexibility, and creativity in a patient. This perhaps surprising characterization is not exaggerated. Try it out for yourself as applied to a dedicated therapeutic experience with a patient. A clinician who is truly *involved* with his or her patient is likely to have an experience of discovery that defies and expands expectation. *Key to this shift may be the uniqueness that results from bringing incongruent items (variables) together to guide one's clinical work.* Also, there are significant concomitants of awe. These can be summarized as reduced focus on oneself and enhanced attention and empathic concern for one's patient, as well as improved flexibility and creativity in one's clinical work (see Chapter 6 for elaboration).

Concluding Thoughts

50

Introduction

In this chapter, we consolidate our clinical model to reflect our paradigm shift. "Clinical complexity" consists not just of numbers, types, and magnitudes of variables, but also when and how during treatment they interrelate. These factors work together to create a clinical tapestry that constantly evolves, both within the patient and in interaction with the environment. Unexpected developments may add further complexity to the clinical situation. Solomon's and Michael's presentations (below) are replete with these typically unbidden and often unnoticed intrusions.

Solomon (The Impact of Unexpected Life Events)

Solomon was a transgendered male, originally a female. He was comfortable with his revised identity and didn't like to think about his (previously female) breasts. He was well accepted by his friends, family, and partner. Solomon worked in construction, fit-positive-healthy. So, it did not seem like a big deal to him when at first his right breast started to ache. Exercise would fix it.

But there is more. There was the disapproving cultural environment, an encounter with which was always a bit shocking for Solomon. Oh, and what about his painful right knee, a result of kneeling all day on hard surfaces. Unexpected and unwelcomed then was a diagnosis of recurrent right sided breast cancer. Alas, Solomon's aching right breast, "an incidental observation," turns out to be only the tip of an ominous iceberg.

Michael (Completing His Diagnosis)

Why not take each item in a case description in sequence, as it comes up?

Because, it generally doesn't work that way in "real" clinical life. Complicating events occur often unannounced and/or unnoticed. That fact was illustrated as we identified the jagged points of clinical discovery in Michael's treatment (Chapter 48). But there are also the permutations, the way variables and events are positioned in time and space and influence one another.

Michael discovered one of my books at a time when he was feeling overwhelmed by problems at work as well as the stress of worrying that another psychiatric treatment could fail. (It would be the tenth in an unrelenting series of failures.) Indeed, Michael was looking for clarity about how to move on with his hobbled life. The timing of his finding my book provided a hoped-for blueprint for overcoming this pattern of repeated failures. But, other complicating factors were at work as well, including his possibly sensing my (SAF) eagerness to take on another patient. Added were legal difficulties which Michael sought to keep private, wanting to avoid exposure associated with involvement with another psychiatrist.

Our Paradigm Shift

Our paradigm shift refers to the recognition of the multitude of evolving, component variables in a clinical situation. These are continually brought together, creating new, often more complicated variable configurations as treatment progresses. Newly created variables may, for example, include elusive individual variables, obscure clinical categories, and/or contributing factors not typically considered clinically relevant.

Retrospective

Here we are at the last moments in the book. You must be curious about the fate of the players in our various dramas. Some of them have succeeded and others failed.

SAF initially was impressed by Michael. As SAF worked to understand Michael, a different Michael began to emerge. He progressively became dismissive, unwilling, or unable to respond to SAF's entreaties. Interpersonal probing followed, with SAF seeking consultation from a colleague to understand why his efforts with Michael were failing. Ultimately, SAF's questioning, including his seeking information from Michael's previous treaters slowly produced a new picture of Michael. It was devoid of the embellishments of Michael's character that SAF had inadvertently introduced previously.

Omar, the refugee from the Middle East, failed to pay his bill repeatedly. In fact he probably had no intention of paying it. This acknowledgement leaves a small hole in my heart because I (SAF) liked and felt sorry for him. Isolated from his family, Omar had little choice about whether to work with an American psychiatrist. That treatment was further crippled by his fear that he might be discovered and reported to authorities at home, leaving him unable to talk about the torture he had been through during war.

Complicating the situation immeasurably with Omar was his surreptitious drug seeking. This was a "#1" variable that I recognized only over time. It was a while before I realized that his story about "requiring" methylphenidate was fabricated. I would have liked to believe that this behavior reflected personal distress, and perhaps it did. He claimed that it was hard for him to get his "medication" as an unnaturalized US resident with only a "green card" to legitimize himself.

My experience with Omar was a contrast to that with Nafi. Nafi at first was obdurate and anything but insightful. He only gradually became a genuine collaborator. The women with whom he was involved were Akane and Artemis, Nafi ultimately was so distraught at his failures with them that he almost required psychiatric hospitalization. Nafi was a brilliant economist according to others who knew him well, but he used terrible judgment with women. At first, he provided a home for each woman, letting her take advantage of him. While I worked hard to engage him, it took over a year before Nafi could really trust me. Prior to that, there was endless dismissiveness not just on his part but ultimately on mine as well based on my frustrations with engaging him.

A profound shift in the quality of our interaction began silently as I attempted to comprehend Nafi's despair. He had just been through a period of intense anguish about losing Akane. His plan for recovery was to cease trying to reestablish his life in the United States and return to live with his mother in Pakistan. He had just about given up the idea of making it on his own in a new country. His only proposal about how to add meaning to his life was to study and learn Mandarin Chinese. Learning this language he asserted could help him in business. Nonetheless, there were no real glimmers of optimism, only despair.

But, out of nowhere, there was a silver lining. Nafi's choice to study Mandarin Chinese and his facility with language forced him into the company of strangers, mostly women. This windfall began to enrich his arid personal experience. He didn't acknowledge at first that there was hope. Everything remained glum. But even in his despair he began to make friends and he started to "warm up" with me, allowing me to "really" get to know him.

We began to talk. He showed me a new, more introspective side of himself. Remarkably, we began to bond. I was shocked at finding in him someone with whom I could relate and even admire. Considering the background of our relationship, this was an experience of amazement for me (a variety of the experience of awe), nothing short of it.

Over the next six months Nafi changed. He became as attentive to others as he had claimed he was capable of being. He had always insisted that he was uniquely capable of being responsive to the needs of others but had never been able to show it. In his involvement with his adult classmates, he was given that opportunity, a new role for someone who had always been taken care of and had been personally isolated. My narrow view of Nafi began to yield. I could "feel" him and apparently he could "feel" me.

What Is the "Old" Paradigm and What Is It Being Replaced By?

Some of the following will be repetitious but we think appropriate for ending this book. Ordinarily, Jennifer would simply be seen as a cranky, elderly woman. She had a lot of money but was withholding of it in ways paralleling her tightness with emotions. Her main psychological problem was anxiety. Reorienting our clinical paradigm moves our perspective from a conventional one based on a limited number of relatively static variables (that could be constructed, for example, as a clinical algorithm) to one emphasizing clinical complexity and the random nature of life events. Jennifer's psychology and pathology are schematized in the "path" diagram already presented (Chapter 47). With this you have a multidimensional rendering of a person. A human being subject to a multitude of influences originating both internally and externally. These can be represented mathematically using vectors and matrices as well as correlated variables in a path-like analysis. We can use this vantage point to generate abductive clinical hypotheses.

With this shift, Jennifer becomes much more than an elderly woman with a history of cancer. She expands to be a truly multidimensional person. A kaleidoscopic view reveals constellations of variables at work. Picture these variables working together (attracting and repelling) and witness the way they shape one another as they evolve.

That is the picture we want to create, the interacting parts and how they work together. The patient is a living, feeling, complex organism, and the objective is for the clinician to achieve a reasonably precise understanding of that person. Ideally, the clinician and the patient "lose themselves" in this shared experience. The result is likely to be the reshaping of the patient's and even the clinician's "sense of self," potentially yielding a renewed focus around which the treatment can move on. This process is by nature transformational for one or both treatment partners. Nafi has become distinctly more open. Jennifer has developed a new, heartfelt capacity for empathy.

Our paradigm shift is in this direction, with the clinical process recognized as complex and dynamic. Perhaps we need a new name for this paradigm. One proposal is to call it a, "complexity model of clinical practice," reflecting its comprehensive and continually evolving nature.

With that inducement we conclude this book. We invite you to come along with us over time as we move further into the world of clinical complexity.

Index

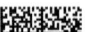